CH00937694

Domestic Violence in Healt
Guide for Healthcare Professions

Parveen Ali • Julie McGarry
Editors

Domestic Violence in Health Contexts: A Guide for Healthcare Professions

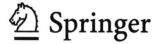 Springer

Editors
Parveen Ali
School of Health Sciences
University of Sheffield
Sheffield
South Yorkshire
UK

Julie McGarry
School of Health Sciences
The University of Nottingham
Queen's Medical Centre
Nottingham
UK

ISBN 978-3-030-29360-4   ISBN 978-3-030-29361-1   (eBook)
https://doi.org/10.1007/978-3-030-29361-1

© Springer Nature Switzerland AG 2020
This work is subject to copyright. All rights are reserved by the Publisher, whether the whole or part of the material is concerned, specifically the rights of translation, reprinting, reuse of illustrations, recitation, broadcasting, reproduction on microfilms or in any other physical way, and transmission or information storage and retrieval, electronic adaptation, computer software, or by similar or dissimilar methodology now known or hereafter developed.
The use of general descriptive names, registered names, trademarks, service marks, etc. in this publication does not imply, even in the absence of a specific statement, that such names are exempt from the relevant protective laws and regulations and therefore free for general use.
The publisher, the authors, and the editors are safe to assume that the advice and information in this book are believed to be true and accurate at the date of publication. Neither the publisher nor the authors or the editors give a warranty, expressed or implied, with respect to the material contained herein or for any errors or omissions that may have been made. The publisher remains neutral with regard to jurisdictional claims in published maps and institutional affiliations.

This Springer imprint is published by the registered company Springer Nature Switzerland AG
The registered company address is: Gewerbestrasse 11, 6330 Cham, Switzerland

Preface

The aim of this book is to provide an introduction for healthcare professionals to the topic of domestic violence and abuse (DVA), which is a complex and multi-faceted phenomenon. In Chap. 1, we begin by highlighting this complexity, for example, in the terminology that is used surrounding DVA and how this is defined within the literature. We also present an overview of the nature and scope of DVA and include some of the main types of abuse, such as physical, psychological, sexual, financial, and coercive control. In Chap. 2, we move beyond the possible manifestations of DVA to present its varied theoretical underpinnings. In this chapter, we introduce the different categories of DVA developed and highlighted within the DVA literature. In Chap. 3, we present details of various classifications or typologies that have been put forward over time to help us understand the complexities of DVA and its various causes, correlations and consequences. There is a growing recognition of the importance of effective management of DVA within healthcare settings acknowledging that there are numerous areas of healthcare practice (including minor injury units and sexual health clinics) where those who have experienced DVA may present. In Chap. 4, Michaela Rogers focuses on several settings where practitioners may encounter presentations of DVA, such as general practice, midwifery and antenatal care, emergency department and mental health settings. In Chap. 5, Kathryn Hinsliff-Smith examines the debates and evidence surrounding DVA, routine enquiry and the support mechanisms that are in place to support those working in clinical practice. In Chap. 6, Caroline Bradbury-Jones and colleagues explore the key issues for children within the context of DVA and emphasise the importance of ensuring that they are always considered in cases of suspected or known DVA. In Chap. 7, Sarah Wydall explores DVA among older people and provides guidance for health professionals on how to respond effectively to DVA in cases involving people aged 60 years and over. Many communities face marginalisation and social exclusion, and, subsequently, they can be considered hidden or hard to reach. These communities are often absent from mainstream discourse, research, policy and practice because of the processes of invisibilisation or systemic exclusion because of practices or structures that uphold systemic exclusion. In Chap. 8, Michaela Rogers considers some of these hard-to-reach communities who can be invisible in policy, practice and research concerning DVA. In Chap. 9, we consider the centrality of multi-agency working among those who encounter victim-survivors of DVA. We set our discussion within the context of the real-life serious case review (SCR). Finally, in Chap. 10, we explore the implications for practice and future areas of learning for healthcare professionals who may encounter victim-survivors of DVA in everyday working.

Taken as a whole, we hope that you will find this text helpful as you begin to explore DVA within healthcare contexts.

Sheffield, UK   Parveen Ali
Nottingham, UK   Julie McGarry

Acknowledgement

We would like to thank so many people who have made this book possible. We couldn't have done it without them.

Contents

About the Authors

Parveen Ali, PhD, MScN, SFHEA, FRSA works as a senior lecturer at the University of Sheffield. She has been associated with the University for more than 10 years now. She is a Registered Nurse, Registered Midwife (Pakistan), Registered Nurse Teacher, senior fellow of Higher Education Academy and a fellow of the Royal Society of Arts, Manufactures and Commerce. She is an associate editor of *Nursing Open* (a Wiley journal) and editorial board member of *Journal of Advanced Nursing* and *Journal of Interpersonal Violence*.

She completed her PhD from the University of Sheffield and her MScN and BScN from the Aga Khan University, Karachi, Pakistan. Her research focuses on gender-based violence, domestic abuse, inequalities in health related to gender and ethnicity and healthcare professionals' preparation. She is a mixed method researcher and has led and contributed to many different projects over the past decade.

She is a recipient of various awards including Mary Seacole Leadership Award, Sigma's Emerging Nurse Researcher Award for Europe and Pakistani Diaspora Achievement Award. She also leads a health programme on a community radio station to raise awareness about different health issues. Parveen serves on various grant awarding bodies and research ethics committees in the UK and other countries. She also loves to contribute to the development of healthcare professionals nationally and internationally to ensure healthcare professionals are prepared to meet the needs of individuals, families, communities and healthcare systems in this changing world.

Caroline Bradbury-Jones, RN, HV, MA, PhD is a registered nurse, midwife and public health nurse. She holds a position as reader in Nursing at the University of Birmingham, UK, where she leads the Risk, Abuse and Violence Research Programme. Her research focuses primarily on violence against women and girls. Her funded research focuses on interventions to improve health professionals' responses to gender-based violence. A large part of her work is undertaken in Africa, where the focus is on community-based approaches to tackling abuse and violence.

Elize Freeman is service development lead and family wellbeing practitioner with Dewis Choice, an innovative participatory action research project, integrating justice, criminal and civil options and wellbeing support for victim survivors of domestic abuse aged 60 years and over. She is an accredited independent domestic violence advisor (IDVA), independent sexual violence advisor (ISVA) and group five accredited gender-based violence service manager on the Wales National Framework, with expertise in service design and delivery for people experiencing domestic violence perpetrated by intimate partners and adult family members. She is an experienced trainer, designing and delivering developmental workshops to social work and safeguarding professionals in partnership with Social Care Wales and the Office of the Older People's Commissioner Wales and specialist practitioner training for Independent Domestic Violence Advisors working with older victim survivors for the UK's national training provider Safelives. She has a BSc (Hons) in digital technology and social science, concentrated on social policy and equality. She is passionate about equality of access to resources and support for victim survivors of domestic abuse and has training in counselling support and family work and is a dementia champion for the Alzheimer's Society UK.

Kathryn Hinsliff-Smith, PhD, MA, PGCE, BA (Hons) is a senior research fellow at De Montfort University, Leicester, UK, based in the Faculty of Health and Life Sciences, is a social scientist with a specialism around qualitative methodologies and is a trained teacher with a background in further and higher education in the UK. She has been involved in evidence-based healthcare for the past decade and completed a Masters in Research Methods and doctoral work on preregistration nurses education. She is actively engaged in research that relates to social justice and health inequalities and has conducted work around gender-based violence. Her expertise relates to research conducted with older populations, in particular their healthcare needs, and survivors of domestic violence. She has been engaged on research grants with international collaborators in Brazil, South Africa and Kenya.

She completed a Joanna Briggs Institute (JBI) systematic review programme and since 2015 is an accredited JBI trainer and reviewer. She has published a number of systematic reviews and presented widely at conference.

She is an associate editor for *Nurse Education in Practice*, a leading international journal which publishes work directly related to education of the workforce, and is a member of the two UK research groups on gender-based violence housed within Nottingham and DMU Universities.

Cathy Humphreys, PhD is co-director of the Safer Families Centre of Research Excellence and professor of Social Work at the University of Melbourne, Australia. She is also co-chair for the Melbourne Alliance to End Violence Against Women and Their Children (MAEVe). She leads a significant programme of research in the areas of domestic and family violence and out-of-home care that has been sustained since 2006 and supported through eight Australian Research Council grants and numerous other grants from government, philanthropy and community sector organisations. She worked as a social work practitioner in the mental health, domestic violence and children, youth and families sector for 16 years before becoming a social work academic. She worked at the University of Warwick in the UK for 12 years prior to returning to Australia.

Julie McGarry, DHSci, MMedSci, BA (Hon) is a registered nurse (RN) in Adult and Mental Health Fields of Practice, Nursing and Midwifery Council Registered Nurse Teacher and Associate Professor in the School of Health Sciences with expertise and professional background in the field of adult and mental health nursing, safeguarding (adults and children), gender-based violence and intimate partner violence/domestic violence and abuse with a focus towards survivors' experiences—the impact on health and wellbeing alongside the development of effective multi-agency (health/social care/criminal justice) responses. She has led a number of externally funded research initiatives, working with international, national and local agencies in the UK in the development of safeguarding and domestic violence services for children and families and survivors of abuse. She also has a well-established background in participant-led research exploring effective approaches to domestic violence identification and management through co-production of arts-based narrative projects with survivors of female genital mutilation (FGM) and DVA. Her current research includes healthcare responses to sexual violence in South Africa—funded through British Council Global Challenge Funds. She has initiated multi-agency collaborative scholarly partnerships on both international and national levels through leading the successful inception and as chair of the *Integrated Domestic Violence and Abuse Research Group* within the Social Futures Centre of Excellence, Institute of Mental Health.

Anita Morris, PhD is a qualified social worker and currently works in state government in Victoria, Australia. Her current role is director, Statewide Hubs Policy and Design, which has responsibility for model development of The Orange Door, an integrated practice and co-location model of family violence and child and family response that is a recommendation arising from the Royal Commission into Family Violence (2016). Also, she is undertaking domestic violence research with children in conjunction with the Safer Families Centre at the University of Melbourne of which Professor Cathy Humphreys is a co-director.

Michaela Rogers, PhD, MA, PgCAP, BA (Hons) is a registered social worker (HCPC) and senior lecturer in Social Work at the University of Sheffield. She has a professional and academic background in the field of social work and social care. Her practice experience ranges from statutory social work in safeguarding children and young people to voluntary sector management and frontline positions working with groups of vulnerable people (e.g. women and children escaping domestic abuse). Her research spans the areas of social care, social justice, equality and diversity, safeguarding, interpersonal abuse and gender-based violence. These projects typically aim to explore social problems in terms of everyday experiences or assess the impact of service delivery or specific policy initiatives. For example, her work on gender-based violence and domestic abuse has a focus towards the experiences of marginalised groups (LGBTQ communities and older people) exploring the barriers and enablers to accessing support. Her current projects examine social norming approaches with young people in prevention programmes which promote healthy relationships.

Dana Sammut, RN is a registered nurse and part-time teaching associate at the University of Birmingham. Her research interests include gender-based violence and healthcare education. Since her undergraduate degree, she has worked closely with Dr. Caroline Bradbury-Jones on a number of projects including research papers, a local service evaluation report and a GBV e-learning resource for healthcare students.

Sarah Wydall is head of the Centre for Age, Gender and Social Justice at Aberystwyth University, Wales. For the last 7 years, she has undertaken research in the area of domestic violence and abuse across the life course. Her recent projects use community-based participatory action research to design and implement a service for older victim survivors in Wales, England and Scotland across the life course. The projects adopt prospective longitudinal research to capture the lived experiences of victim-survivors at different stages in the help-seeking journey.

In 2016, she won the Audrey Jones Memorial Award for Feminist Scholarship for 'Undertaking Transformative Research with Victim-Survivors in Wales: Dewis Choice, A Story of Feminist Praxis'. She is also a member of the International Network Addressing Filial Violence established by Monash and Oxford Universities, given her knowledge on older people and domestic abuse. She has also acted in an advisory capacity on a number of working groups including work on older people and domestic homicide for standing together against domestic violence and abuse. She has written guidance for the Welsh Government and the Older People's Commissioner for Wales on domestic violence and abuse and has delivered training for Safelives on older people and domestic homicide.

Introduction to Domestic Violence and Abuse Within Healthcare Contexts

1

Parveen Ali and Julie McGarry

1.1 Introduction

Domestic violence and abuse (DVA) is a significant public health and social care issue which affects millions of individuals and families, across the world. In this first chapter, we will begin to explore the phenomenon of DVA. We will provide an introduction to some of key issues, diversity and complexity that surrounds DVA and how DVA is situated within the wider spectrum of violence and abuse within families. We will then consider why DVA forms an important and integral part of contemporary healthcare practice for all healthcare professionals.

We are all familiar with the word violence, gender based violence and domestic violence, although we don't always stop to consider what these terms actually mean and if there is any overlap between the different concepts. Let's take this opportunity to look at the word "violence" and what it means first. The World Health Organization (WHO) (1996) defines violence as *"the intentional use of physical force or power, threatened or actual, against oneself, another person, or against a group or community, that either results in or has a high likelihood of resulting in injury, death, psychological harm, mal-development or deprivation"* (p. 4). As mentioned earlier, while violence can affect anyone, girls and women remain to be

P. Ali (✉)
School of Health Sciences, University of Sheffield, Sheffield, UK
e-mail: Parveen.ali@sheffield.ac.uk

J. McGarry
School of Health Sciences, The University of Nottingham, Queen's Medical Centre, Nottingham, UK
e-mail: Julie.McGarry@nottingham.ac.uk; https://institutemh.org.uk/research/centre-for-social-futures/projects/349-research-area-domestic-violence-and-abuse

© Springer Nature Switzerland AG 2020
P. Ali, J. McGarry (eds.), *Domestic Violence in Health Contexts: A Guide for Healthcare Professions*, https://doi.org/10.1007/978-3-030-29361-1_1

major victims of violence in public as well as private sphere and therefore violence is considered a gendered issue.

Other terms that you may have noticed being used within the literature are violence against women (VAW) and gender based violence (GBV), both of which refer to *"any act of gender-based violence that results in, or is likely to result in, physical, sexual or mental harm or suffering to women, including threats of such acts, coercion or arbitrary deprivation of liberty, whether occurring in public or in private life"* (United Nations 1993). VAW can take many different forms, including female infanticide, female genital mutilation, child marriage, grooming, trafficking, forced marriage, dowry abuse, honour based violence, rape, sexual assault, stalking, harassment, street violence, domestic abuse (DVA), and intimate partner violence (IPV). While GBV and VAW encompass every form of violence and abuse against girls and women, a major portion of such abuse happens in the context of private life and individual relationships and therefore it is known as DVA.

DVA is defined in the United Kingdom (UK) as *"any incident or pattern of incidents of controlling, coercive, threatening behaviour, violence or abuse between those aged 16 or over who are, or have been, intimate partners or family members regardless of gender or sexuality. The abuse can encompass, but is not limited to psychological, physical, sexual, financial or emotional"* (National Institute for Health and Care Excellence 2016). This definition also encompasses acts of "honour" based violence, female genital mutilation (FGM) [cutting], and forced marriage. DVA in itself is a complex issue and can manifest itself in several forms, including child abuse, elder abuse, and IPV.

From the description above, you may have gathered that there is no single definition of DVA within the literature and that the terms DVA, IPV, and family violence can be quite confusing and many people use them interchangeably. Other terms to refer to same behaviour may also include domestic abuse, domestic violence, intimate partner abuse, partner violence, partner abuse, etc. They are not actually the same thing and there are distinctions between them. DVA is a broad term that encompasses a range of abuse and violence that occurs within a domestic context. The perpetrator might be a partner or other family member. This is reflected in the definition by the UK government provided above. You may also notice, as you read around the subject, that some people think that the term domestic violence is related to the use of physical force and that the term domestic abuse is related to use of psychological abuse and controlling behaviour. However, both terms are used interchangeably to refer to the same behaviour. In this book, we use the term 'domestic violence and abuse' (DVA) as we prefer this broader term. However, for the most part we focus on intimate partner violence (IPV) because that has been our main area of research and it is the most common form of violence within a domestic context. In addition, terms violence and abuse will be used interchangeably.

It is well established that DVA affects a significant number of individuals and families worldwide and intersects cultural, religious, gender, and ethnic boundaries. It can occur in marital, cohabiting, heterosexual as well as same sex relationships (Ali et al. 2016; Baker et al. 2013). While it should be acknowledged that men, women as well as transgender people in straight, gay, or lesbian relationships can all perpetrate and experience DVA, it is important to recognise that DVA is experienced disproportionately by women and perpetrated predominantly by men. The abuse that women experience is repeated, systematic, more severe and more likely to result in injury or death. Men, as current or former intimate partners, remain the most common perpetrators of partner violence.

Time to Reflect
As a starting point, we would ask you to think about the ways in which you may have encountered the term 'domestic violence and abuse' so far. This may have included reading academic texts or articles and/or wider media reports. How do you define domestic violence and abuse? What does it mean to you and are you aware of any other terms used to describe the same phenomenon?

You may wish to make some brief notes and return to these as you continue to read and access the resources within this book. As you read the different chapters, consider if you would change anything about your initial views.

1.2   Forms of DVA

DVA can take many forms as indicated in Fig. 1.1. The most common forms include physical, sexual, and psychological abuse (WHO 2002). Financial or economic abuse and social abuse are some other categories identified; however, it is not clear if these subcategories and especially the category relating to social abuse actually exist as separate dimensions of DVA. Coercive control is another form of abuse, more recently acknowledged in its own entity—previously it was largely subsumed within psychological abuse. Individuals may be exposed to one or more forms of abuse at one time (Devries et al. 2013; World Health Organization 2013). It is also

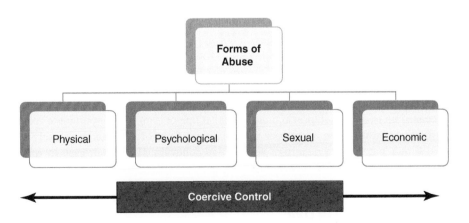

Fig. 1.1 Forms of domestic violence and abuse

worthy of note that you may also come across additional categories of abuse and as such our list is not meant to be exhaustive.

Let's now look at each of these types of abuse in more detail:

Physical violence or abuse refers to the use of physical force to inflict pain, injury, or physical suffering to the victim. Example of abusive acts includes slapping, beating, kicking, pinching, biting, pushing, shoving, dragging, stabbing, spanking, scratching, hitting with a fist or something else that could hurt, burning, choking, threatening or using a gun, knife or any other weapon (García-Moreno et al. 2005).

Sexual violence or abuse refers to "any sexual act, attempt to obtain a sexual act, unwanted sexual comments or advances, or acts to traffic, or otherwise directed, against a person's sexuality using coercion, by any person, regardless of their relationship to the victim, in any setting, including but not limited to home and work" (Jewkes et al. 2002, p. 149). In the context of DVA, sexual abuse refers to physically force a partner, to have sexual intercourse, forcing a partner to do something that they found degrading or humiliating (García-Moreno et al. 2005), harming them during sex or forcing them to have sex without protection (World Health Organization 2014).

Psychological violence or abuse refers to the use of various behaviours intended to humiliate and control another individual in public or private. Examples of psychological violence include verbal abuse, name calling, constantly criticising, blackmailing, saying something or doing something to make the other person feel embarrassed, threats to beat women or children, monitoring and restricting movements, restricting access to friends and family, restricting economic independence and access to information, assistance or other resources and services such as education or health services (Follingstad and DeHart 2000; WHO 2002).

Financial or Economical Abuse refers to controlling a person's ability to acquire, use, and maintain their own money and resources. An abuser may prevent a woman from working to earn her own money (not letting her go to work; sabotaging job interviews, taking the welfare benefits she is entitled to), using their money without consent, building up debts in her name, damaging her property and possessions, withholding maintenance payments, etc.

Coercive control is another specific form of IPV/DVA which has now become a reportable offence in some countries especially the UK. It is defined as any act or a pattern of acts of assault, threats, humiliation and intimidation or other abuse that is used to harm, punish, or frighten their victim (United Kingdom Home Office 2013). At times, coercive control is used in the absence of physical and sexual abuse and is more difficult to spot. It is now a criminal offence in some countries such as the UK and if the abuser is found guilty of coercively controlling the victim, they can be sentenced up to 5 years in prison, made to pay a fine or both. It is important to recognise that victims often experience more than one form of DVA and it is rarely a one-off incident, but is a pattern of abusive and controlling behaviour used by one person against the other.

1.3   Prevalence of DVA

Knowing the exact prevalence of DVA in any country is challenging; however, data collection is getting better every day owing to more focus on the issue by national and international organisations in each country. Let's look at the prevalence of DVA in the UK and other countries. According to the Crime Survey for England and Wales (CSEW 2018), an estimated 2.0 million adults aged 16–59 years experienced DVA in the year ending March 2018, equating to a prevalence rate of approximately 6%. Women were around twice as likely to have experienced DVA than men (7.9% compared with 4.2%). This equates to an estimated 1.3 million female victims and 695,000 male victims (UK Office for National Statistics 2018). Figure 1.2 below provides an overview of DVA experienced by adults aged 16–59 years, by sex and compares the rate between 2005 and 2018. The figure clearly highlights a slight decrease in the prevalence of DVA overtime, though these findings should be read with caution as a number of researchers have highlighted the potential limitations with current measurement and reporting of DVA which, it is argued, does not accurately capture the context or impact of harm (Myhill 2017).

We know that DVA affects all communities and countries; however, estimating the prevalence within and between countries is difficult due to inconsistent definitions, under-reporting, and a lack of epidemiological studies. The psychological, intimate, and private nature of the abuse means that it is often not reported. Victims may not want to report it or may not recognise their experience as abuse. There are inconsistencies in reporting, recording, and defining DVA. To deal with this issue, the World Health Organization sponsored a multi-country study involving ten countries, including Bangladesh, Brazil, Ethiopia, Japan, Namibia, Peru, Samoa, Serbia and Montenegro, Thailand, and Tanzania using standardised population-based household surveys (García-Moreno et al. 2005). Their findings based on interviews from 24,097 women aged 15–49 years revealed a lifetime prevalence of physical and sexual DVA ranging from 15 to 71%. The proportion of women who had ever experienced physical violence ranged from 13% in Japan to 61% in Peru province. Lifetime prevalence of sexual violence experienced by women ranged from 6% in Japan to 59% in Peru (2005). The study also attempted to identify the prevalence of physical violence

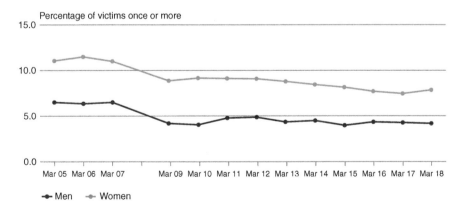

Fig. 1.2 Prevalence of domestic abuse for adults aged 16–59 years, by sex: England and Wales, year ending March 2005 to year ending March 2018. (Source: SEW, Office for National Statistics. No data point is available for the year ending March 2008 because comparable questions on stalking, an offence that makes up the domestic abuse category, were not included in that year)

according to severity. Acts such as slapping, pushing, and shoving were classified as moderate violent acts, whereas dragging, kicking, threatening with a weapon, or using a weapon against women were classified as severe violent acts. The proportion of ever-partnered women who experienced severe physical violence ranged from 4% in Japan to 49% in Peru. Physical violence only or both physical and sexual violence were identified as the most common form of abuse experienced by women. Thirty to 56% of women reported both physical and sexual violence. While women experience violence at a higher rate, in many cases DVA accounts for majority of women's experiences of violence.

During the past decade, a number of countries attempted to collect data about VAW and DVA, especially with the help of Demographic Health Survey (DHS). The findings of various surveys estimate that 35% of women, worldwide, have experienced physical and/or sexual violence at some point in their life. Though, some national studies maintain that up to 70% of women have experienced physical and/or sexual DVA in their lifetime (United Nations 2015). Figures from DHS suggest that the proportion of women experiencing physical and/or sexual violence in their lifetime ranged from 6 to 64%. Prevalence was generally higher in Africa than in other regions, with one quarter of countries in the region reporting lifetime prevalence of at least 50%. Prevalence was lower across Asia, Latin America and the Caribbean and Oceania with maximum prevalence levels of around 40%. For physical and/or sexual abuse experienced in the 12 months prior to the survey, prevalence ranged from 5 to 44%. The rates of prevalence of DVA in the past 12 months were often similar to lifetime prevalence (Fig. 1.3).

In the Europe, the European Union Agency for Fundamental Rights conducted an EU-wide survey in 2014 (European Union Agency for Fundamental Rights 2014) and the findings suggest a lifetime prevalence of physical and/or sexual abuse ranged from 13 to 32% in Denmark and Latvia. Prevalence of DVA experienced in the past 12 months was generally lower and ranged between 2 and 6%. Rates of lifetime physical and/or sexual abuse were highest in Oceania, with prevalence reaching over 60% in a number of countries in the region. Experience in the past 12 months was typically much lower than the lifetime (Fig. 1.4).

The proportion of women experiencing psychological abuse in their lifetime ranged from 7 to 68%, whereas the prevalence of psychological abuse experienced in the 12 months prior to the survey ranged from 6 to 40%. Experience in the past 12 months was generally similar to lifetime experience in Africa, Asia, and Oceania; however, in Latin America and the Caribbean recent experience was considerably lower than a lifetime. In EU countries, the proportion of women experiencing psychological abuse at least once in their lives ranged from 31 to 60%.

Economic abuse is difficult to define and varies significantly in various settings due to differences in the cultural context and circumstances. Available evidence suggests the life prevalence of economic abuse as 25%, whereas prevalence of economic abuse in last 12 months, prior to the survey, was reported to be 17% (United Nations 2015). We also know that women who experience physical and sexual abuse are more likely to experience economic abuse. This could take the form of the husband taking their wife's earned or saved money from them or refusing to financially support them (United Nations 2015).

Fig. 1.3 Proportion of ever-partnered women aged 15–49 years experiencing intimate partner physical and/or sexual violence at least once in their lifetime and in the last 12 months, 1995–2013. (United Nations, 2015. *The World's Women 2015: Trends and Statistics*. New York: United Nations, Department of Economic and Social Affairs, Statistics Division. Sales No. E.15.XVII.8)

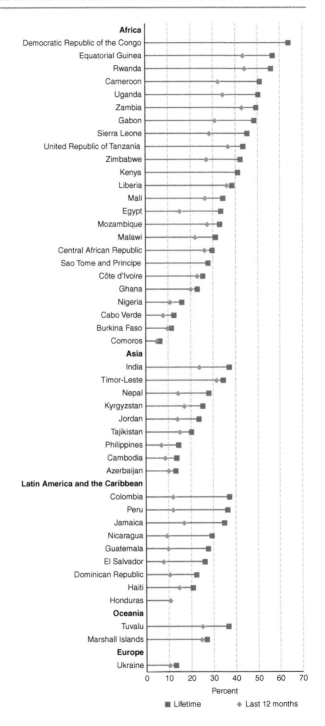

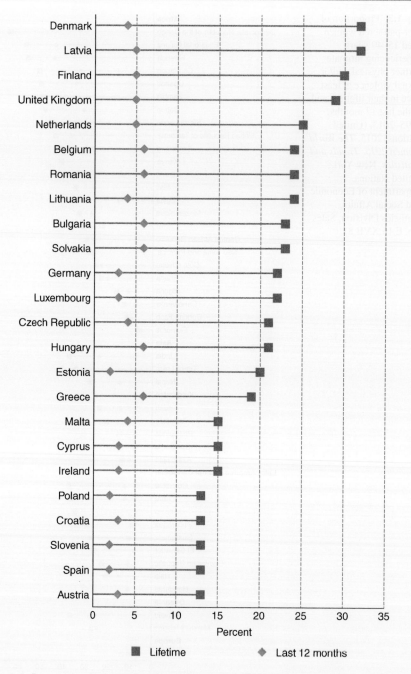

Fig. 1.4 Proportion of ever-partnered women aged 18–74 years experiencing intimate partner physical and/or sexual violence at least once in their lifetime and in the last 12 months, European countries, 2012. (United Nations, 2015. *The World's Women 2015: Trends and Statistics*. New York: United Nations, Department of Economic and Social Affairs, Statistics Division. Sales No. E.15. XVII.8. European Union Agency for Fundamental Rights, Violence against Women: An EU-wide survey, 2014. (European Union Agency for Fundamental Rights 2014))

1.4   Violence During Pregnancy

DVA does not stop in pregnancy but in fact for many women it starts or escalates during pregnancy. According to the findings of the WHO multi-country study on women's health and domestic violence against women, the prevalence of physical violence during pregnancy ranged between 1% in Japan city and 28% in Peru Province, with the majority of sites ranging between 4 and 12% (García-Moreno et al. 2005). Similar findings were reported from DHS and the International Violence against Women Survey, which found prevalence rates for DVA during pregnancy between 2% in Australia, Denmark, Cambodia, and Philippines and 13.5% in Uganda, with the majority ranging between 4 and 9% (Devries et al. 2010). Other evidence suggests a higher prevalence of DVA in various countries, including Egypt (32%), India (28%), Saudi Arabia (21%), and Mexico (11%) (Campbell et al. 2004). Another review of clinical studies from Africa reported prevalence rates of 23–40% for physical, 3–27% for sexual, and 25–49% for psychological violence during pregnancy (Shamu et al. 2011). Figure 1.5 shows DHS data

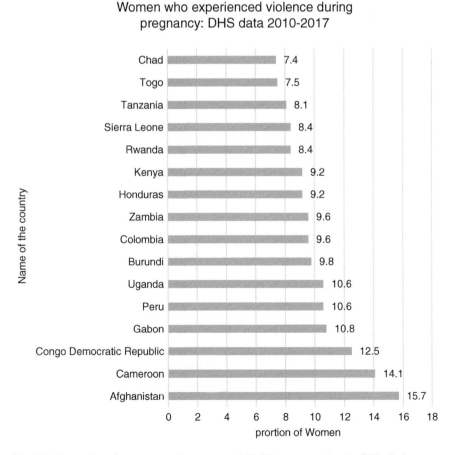

Fig. 1.5 Proportion of ever-partnered women aged 18–74 years experiencing DVA during pregnancy. (Developed by authors using data from Demographic Health Survey)

about women experience of DVA in pregnancy. It shows 17 countries with higher rates of DVA reported during pregnancy, ranging from 7.4% in Chad to 15.7% in Afghanistan.

1.5   Violence Against Men

While, as we noted earlier in this chapter, women remain the main victims of DVA, it is now recognised that men can also be victims of DVA where violence is perpetrated by their female partner. The findings of the CSEW (Office of National Statistics 2018) suggest that an estimated 2.2 million men aged 16–59 had experienced DVA since the age of 16. Table 1.1, provided below, presents statistics on the proportion of women victims of DVA alongside the proportion of women perpetrator of DVA. It clearly highlights that the number of women experiencing DVA is much higher than the number of women perpetrating DVA. As shown there, the only country for which the number of women perpetrator was higher than women victims of violence was the Philippines (2013) where the prevalence of women perpetrated violence against men (16%) was only slightly higher than violence perpetrated by men against women (13%). Some studies also include men's self-reported experiences of violence. Here again, reported rates of physical violence by men against women are higher than those of physical violence by women against men. More research is needed to explore the true extent of violence against men and violence perpetrated by women against men.

1.6   DVA and Health Impacts

DVA is associated with serious psychological as well as physical consequences for not only the victim, but others in the family such as children. We know that approximately 42% of women who experience physical or sexual abuse sustain injuries as a result (World Health Organisation 2013).

The examples of minor physical consequences may include cuts, punctures, bruises, and bites. Severe injuries may result in permanent disability (e.g. loss of limb, hearing loss, damage to teeth). Victims of DVA report higher rates of poor health, compromised ability to walk, pain, vaginal discharge, loss of memory, dizziness, and self-harm compared to those who do not. Other examples of the impact of sexual abuse include unwanted pregnancy, miscarriage, sexually transmitted infections (STI), and other gynaecological problems.

Psychological effects of DVA may include fear, depression, low self-esteem, anxiety disorders, depression, headaches, obsessive-compulsive disorder, posttraumatic stress disorder, low self-esteem, disassociation, sleep disorders, shame, guilt, self-mutilation, drug and alcohol abuse, and eating disorders. Psychological consequences may also manifest through psychosomatic symptoms, sexual dysfunction, and eating problems. In addition, DVA can have fatal consequences for

Table 1.1 Proportion of women who report experiencing lifetime intimate partner physical violence, as victims and perpetrators, 2005–2013

	Women victims	Women perpetrators
Developed regions		
Ukraine	12.7	10.9
Republic of Moldova	24.1	7.1
Oceania		
Marshall Islands	22.1	12.0
Tuvalu	33.3	9.7
Latin America and the Caribbean		
Haiti	15.6	4.9
Peru	35.7	8.5
Asia		
Philippines	12.7	15.8
Cambodia	12.8	6.0
Tajikistan	19.5	2.0
Nepal	23.1	3.1
Kyrgyzstan	25.1	4.2
Timor-Leste	33.5	5.5
India	35.1	0.7
Africa		
Comoros	5.6	5.1
Nigeria	14.4	1.7
Cabo Verde	15.7	4.6
Ghana	20.6	7.0
Malawi	21.7	4.1
Côte d'Ivoire	24.6	1.6
Central Africa Republic	25.4	8.8
Zimbabwe	28.8	3.6
Mali	29.8	3.2
Rwanda	30.7	0.9
Mozambique	31.5	3.7
Liberia	35.0	9.5
Kenya	37.0	3.0
United Republic of Tanzania	39.2	2.4
Uganda	42.7	6.6
Sierra Leone	44.2	7.5
Cameroon	44.8	7.4
Gabon	46.2	22.3
Zambia	46.5	9.8
Equatorial Guinea	54.4	21.5

United Nations, 2015. *The World's Women 2015: Trends and Statistics*. New York: United Nations, Department of Economic and Social Affairs, Statistics Division. Sales No. E.15.XVII.8

victims resulting from homicide or suicide (Black 2011). Similar side effects are reported by victims of female perpetrated violence (with exception to gynaecological symptoms) or those in a same sex relationship.

DVA in pregnancy is also been associated with adverse pregnancy outcomes. A US-based study found that pregnancy significantly increases a woman's risk of becoming a victim of domestic homicide and that men who abuse their pregnant partners are very dangerous and more likely to kill them (Campbell 2002). Clearly, the health outcomes of abuse can be both fatal and non-fatal for pregnant women and their children. Nonfatal impacts result from the impact of trauma to a woman's body as well as the physiological effects of stress from current or past abuse on foetal growth and development. In addition to the non-fatal health outcomes that any victim can experience, for women in pregnancy, there are additional impacts, including: higher rates of preterm labour and stillbirth; placental abruption; low birth weight; other infections and complications (Coker et al. 2012). The strongest risk factors for developing antenatal mental illness have constantly been found to include the existence of DVA as well as other factors, including a history of psychiatric illness, low socioeconomic status, and insufficient social support (Howard et al. 2014; Moncrieff 2018).

1.7 Help Seeking Behaviour

It is important for healthcare professionals to understand that disclosing abusive experiences and seeking help can be very difficult and challenging. Evidence based on DHS surveys conducted between 2014 and 2018 suggest that proportion of women who sought help from family, friends, or institutions such as health services and the police ranged from 9.7% in Tajikistan (2017) to over 54% in Tanzania (2015–2016). In the majority of countries, less than 40% of the women who experienced DVA sought help of any sort. Among those who did, most looked to family and friends. Only a small proportion of women sought help from police. In almost all countries with available data, the percentage of women who sought help from the police was less than 10%. Similarly, the proportion of those sought help from healthcare professionals remained less than 6% as shown in Fig. 1.6. This highlights difficulties associated with disclosing and seeking help from services. There are many different barriers which include lack of awareness of or actual lack of services; lack of accessibility to services due to linguistic, cultural, physical, or financial barriers; fear of repercussions by perpetrator or family and community members; shame or embarrassment; the potential impact on women's custody of children; the feeling that no one could help; and wanting to keep the incident private.

Summary Points
This chapter aimed to provide an overview of DVA, forms of DVA, its prevalence and health impacts. The important points from the chapter are summarised below.

• DVA is a major social and public health issue, and millions of women regardless of income, education, age, or other characteristics experience DVA in its various forms.

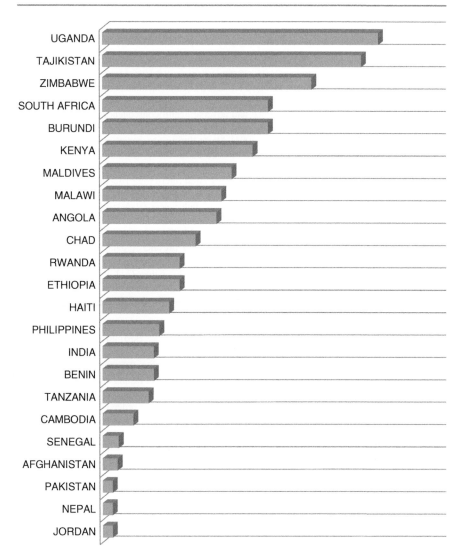

Fig. 1.6 Proportion of women aged 15–49 years who experienced DVA and sought help from healthcare professionals, 2014–2018. (Developed by authors using data from Demographic Health Survey)

- DVA has serious consequences for not only the victims and these include short- and long-term physical, mental, and emotional health problems.
- While men can also be victims of DVA, intensity, frequency, and severity of abuse experienced by women are much worse.
- Disclosing DVA experiences and seeking help from appropriate sources is not easy and the number of women seeking support from appropriate professionals and organisations including the police and healthcare professionals remains very low.

References

Ali PA, Dhingra K, McGarry J (2016) A literature review of intimate partner violence and its clas-
    sifications. Aggress Violent Behav 31:16–25. https://doi.org/10.1016/j.avb.2016.06.008
Baker NL, Buick JD, Kim SR, Moniz S, Nava KL (2013) Lessons from examining same-sex inti-
    mate partner violence. Sex Roles 69(3–4):182–192
Black MC (2011) Intimate partner violence and adverse health consequences: implications for
    clinicians. Am J Lifestyle Med. https://doi.org/10.1177/1559827611410265
Campbell J, Garcia-Moreno C, Sharps P (2004) Abuse during pregnancy in industrialized and
    developing countries. Violence Against Women 10(7):770–789
Campbell J, Jones AS, Dienemann J, Kub J, Schollenberger J, O'Campo P et al (2002) Intimate
    partner violence and physical health consequences. Arch Intern Med 162(10):1157–1163
Coker AL, Follingstad D, Garcia LS, Williams CM, Crawford TN, Bush HM (2012) Association of
    intimate partner violence and childhood sexual abuse with cancer-related well-being in women.
    J Womens Health 21(11):1180–1188
Devries KM, Kishor S, Johnson H, Stöckl H, Bacchus LJ, Garcia-Moreno C, Watts C (2010)
    Intimate partner violence during pregnancy: analysis of prevalence data from 19 countries.
    Reprod Health Matters 18(36):158–170
Devries KM, Mak JY, García-Moreno C, Petzold M, Child JC, Falder G et al (2013) The global
    prevalence of intimate partner violence against women. Science 340(6140):1527–1528
European Union Agency for Fundamental Rights (2014) Violence against women: an EU-wide
    survey
Follingstad DR, DeHart DD (2000) Defining psychological abuse of husbands toward wives:
    contexts, behaviors, and typologies. J Interpers Violence 15(9):891–920. https://doi.
    org/10.1177/088626000015009001
García-Moreno C, Jansen HAFM, Ellsberg M, Heise L, Watts C (2005) WHO multi-country study
    on women's health and domestic violence against women: initial results onprevalence, health
    outcomes and women's responses. World Health Organization, Geneva
Howard RC, Khalifa N, Duggan C (2014) Antisocial personality disorder comorbid with bor-
    derline pathology and psychopathy is associated with severe violence in a forensic sample. J
    Forens Psychiatry Psychol 25(6):658–672
Jewkes R, Sen P, Garcia-Moreno C (2002) Sexual violence. In: Krug EG, Dahlberg LL, Mercy
    JA, Zwi AB, Lozano R (eds) World report on violence and health. World Health Organization,
    Geneva, pp 149–181
Moncrieff G (2018) The cyclical and intergenerational effects of perinatal domestic abuse and
    mental health. Br J Midwifery 26(2):85–93
Myhill A (2017) Measuring domestic violence: context is everything. J Gender Based Violence
    1(1):33–44
National Institute for Health and Care Excellence (2016) Domestic violence and abuse: quality
    standard [QS116]. NICE, UK
Office of National Statistics (2018) Domestic abuse: findings from the Crime Survey for England
    and Wales: year ending March 2018. https://www.ons.gov.uk/peoplepopulationandcommu-
    nity/crimeandjustice/articles/domesticabusefindingsfromthecrimesurveyforenglandandwales/
    yearendingmarch2018
Shamu S, Abrahams N, Temmerman M, Musekiwa A, Zarowsky C (2011) A systematic review
    of African studies on intimate partner violence against pregnant women: prevalence and risk
    factors. PLoS One 6(3):e17591
UK Home Office (2013) Domestic violence and abuse. Retrieved from https://www.gov.uk/
    guidance/domestic-violence-and-abuse#history
United Nations (1993) Declaration on the elimination of violence against women. https://www.
    un.org/documents/ga/res/48/a48r104.htm

WHO (1996) Global consultation on violence and health. Violence: a public health priority ((EHA/SPI.POA.2).). WHO, Geneva
WHO (2002) World report on violence and health: Summary. WHO, Geneva
World Health Organisation (2013) Global and regional estimates of violence against women: prevalence and health effects of intimate partner violence and nonpartner sexual violence. WHO, Geneva. http://apps.who.int/iris/bitstream/10665/85239/1/9789241564625_eng.pdf?ua=1
World Health Organization (2013) Global and regional estimates of violence against women: prevalence and health effects of intimate partner violence and non-partner sexual violence. World Health Organization, Geneva
World Health Organization (2014) Health care for women subjected to intimate partner violence or sexual violence: a clinical handbook. World Health Organization, Geneva

Domestic Violence and Abuse: Theoretical Explanation and Perspectives

2

Parveen Ali, Julie McGarry, and Caroline Bradbury-Jones

We have so far provided an overview of domestic violence and abuse (DVA), its definitions, prevalence, and impact. When developing your knowledge and understanding of DVA, you will almost certainly start to question "why and how" DVA occurs. Over the past few decades, a number of theories and frameworks have been proposed to explain the phenomenon of DVA. The aim of this chapter, therefore, is to provide an overview of various explanations to help you understand the issue of DVA from a conceptual and theoretical perspective. The chapter explores common DVA perspectives, including feminist, social learning, ecological, biological, and psychological.

2.1 Feminist Explanations

The feminist movement is not only responsible for bringing the world's attention to the issue of VAW and DVA but also for establishing women's shelters, initiating various batterer intervention and advocacy programmes, and bringing changes in the legal and criminal justice system to make VAW a criminal offence

P. Ali (✉)
School of Health Sciences, The University of Sheffield, Sheffield, UK
e-mail: Parveen.ali@sheffield.ac.uk

J. McGarry
School of Health Sciences, The University of Nottingham, Queen's Medical Centre, Nottingham, UK
e-mail: Julie.McGarry@nottingham.ac.uk; https://institutemh.org.uk/research/centre-for-social-futures/projects/349-research-area-domestic-violence-and-abuse

C. Bradbury-Jones
University of Birmingham, Birmingham, UK

© Springer Nature Switzerland AG 2020
P. Ali, J. McGarry (eds.), *Domestic Violence in Health Contexts: A Guide for Healthcare Professions*, https://doi.org/10.1007/978-3-030-29361-1_2

(McPhail et al. 2007). According to this perspective, DVA is not a private or family matter, but a deeply embedded social problem that has to be addressed by social change. Feminists believe that violence in heterosexual relationships is always perpetrated by men in an attempt to control their female partner, and that women's use of violence is almost always an act of self-defence. Under this perspective, feminist theorists have offered various explanations for DVA, including the cycle of violence, learned helplessness, the battered women syndrome, the power and control wheel, and patriarchy, which are considered below.

2.1.1 Cycles of Violence

The cycle of violence (see Fig. 2.1) is proposed by Walker (1979) with the aim to explain how and why abused women remain in an abusive relationship. The cycle of violence is often predictable and consists of three phases: tension building; abuse or explosion; and honeymoon or remorse forgiveness. In the first phase, tension builds up within the couple and the abuser starts getting frustrated and takes it out on his partner in the form of DVA. Violence could take a variety of forms, including physical, psychological, emotional, or sexual abuse that may last from seconds to days. The abuser then feels relieved, may start resenting his violent attitude towards his partner, and may start apologising. The couple then enjoys a honeymoon period in which the victim-survivor thinks the abuser will change and violence will stop. In some cases, the intensity of violence is decreased or is stopped for some time and the cycle continues (Walker 2006). Constant exposure to a cycle of violence results

Fig. 2.1 The cycle of violence. (Source: Walker, L. (1979). *The battered woman*. New York: Harper & Row)

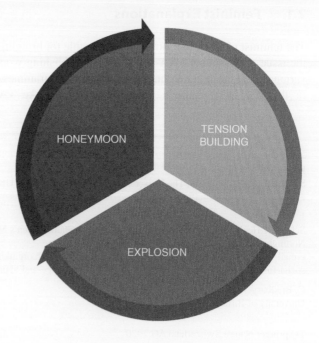

in the development of a feeling of helplessness, reduced decision-making ability, and development of fear (Walker 1979). The victim starts blaming themselves for the abuse and tries to refrain from the situations that could precipitate violence. This theory did not maintain its popularity for long, as women's experiences were not consistent with the theory. Opponents argue that if violence is a result of tension and frustration, why does the abuser only vent his frustration on his partner and not on his work colleagues or other people.

2.1.2   Learned Helplessness

This concept of learned helplessness was first described in the 1960s by a psychologist called Martin Seligman (Seligman and Maier 1967). Seligman and his colleagues conducted a series of controlled experiments by placing dogs in two types of cages. In the first type of cage in conjunction with a conditioned stimulus (a bell), an electric shock was given. The second cage, however, had an area where no shock could be administered. Dogs in the first cage learned to accept the shock and gave up trying to escape, whereas dogs in the second cage learned to run to the shock-proof place. The researchers then placed the dogs from the first cage (shocking cage) to the second cage (with a shockproof place). Interestingly, dogs from the shocking cage did not react to look for an escape route. Seligman and colleagues concluded their observation by asserting that dogs' experiences of repeated, non-contingent, and inescapable shock in the first cage resulted in the development of a feeling of helplessness and inability to control their situation (Overmier and Seligman 1967; Seligman and Maier 1967).

The theory of learned helplessness has been used to explain the behaviour of abused women (Ball and Wyman 1978; Waites 1978; Walker 1977/1978, 1979). Walker (1979) applied this theory to study the behaviour of abused women and concluded that continuous and repeated abuse results in minimising the abused woman's motivation to respond and enforces passiveness. Walker suggested that DVA negatively affects a woman's cognitive ability to perceive success and make them believe that their action cannot generate a positive outcome. As a result, she does not try to leave an abusive relationship. In addition, a feeling of loss of control and helplessness developed in childhood makes individuals, especially women, more vulnerable to physical and sexual abuse in adult life (Walker and Browne 1985). Learned helplessness may also explain why women themselves justify DVA as, for example, the majority of the abused women in WHO's multi-country study (García-Moreno et al. 2005) justified beating under various conditions such as not completing housework effectively, refusing sex, disobeying a husband, or being unfaithful.

Opponents maintain that this theory fails to acknowledge other factors contributing to a woman's decision to stay in an abusive relationship. For instance, social, economic, and cultural reasons such as a fear of retaliation by the husband/partner, inability to financially support herself and children, and a fear of rejection by the family, community and society (Naved et al. 2006). It also does not take into account a woman's conscious effort to minimise violence towards themselves and their children. Victim-survivor women often plan their escape consciously and make arrangements slowly to prepare themselves to leave the relationship in future. Furthermore, manifestations of learned helplessness such as low self-esteem, perceived loss of control, and withdrawal could actually be the effects of abuse.

2.1.3   Battered Women Syndrome

Walker (1979) used the theories of the cycle of violence and learned helplessness to explain the concept or condition of "Battered Women Syndrome", which offered an explanation for a woman's retaliating behaviour. It is basically a sub-type of a condition called posttraumatic stress disorder (PTSD) (Walker 2006). A woman could be classified as battered if she has experienced at least two cycles of violence. The concept has been successfully used in various professional contexts, including clinical interventions, family and custody problems, and as grounds for policy and legal reforms (Craven 2003). The concept has been used in some court cases to defend women who have killed their abusive husbands after spending a lot of time in an abusive relationship (Mossière et al. 2018).

2.1.4   Power and Control

Feminist ideology, resulting from discussions with battered women, contributed to the development of 'the power and control wheel' (see Fig. 2.2). The model was developed in 1980–1981 and was a result of a Domestic Abuse Intervention Project (DAIP) conducted in Duluth in the USA. The model explains the tactics used by abusive men to keep women in submissive positions and to maintain male power and control. The model assumes that no every abusive tactic or behaviour is aimed to keep the women under control and exert male power. The model maintains that the responsibility for abuse and control lies with the abuser and that the overall aim of the interventions should be victim's safety and to hold the abusers accountable for their actions.

2.1.5   Patriarchy

Patriarchy is "an 'umbrella' term for describing men's systemic dominance of women" (Pease 2000: 20). It is characterised by a value and belief system that justifies male dominance and rejects egalitarian structures in the public and private spheres of life. In the public sphere, power is shared by men and in private spheres the senior men exercise power over everyone else in the family, including younger men and boys (Haj-Yahia and Schiff 2007). Therefore, in patriarchal societies, a man is considered and expected to be the head of the family. The use of DVA is an acceptable way of maintaining and exhibiting male dominance. Believers in

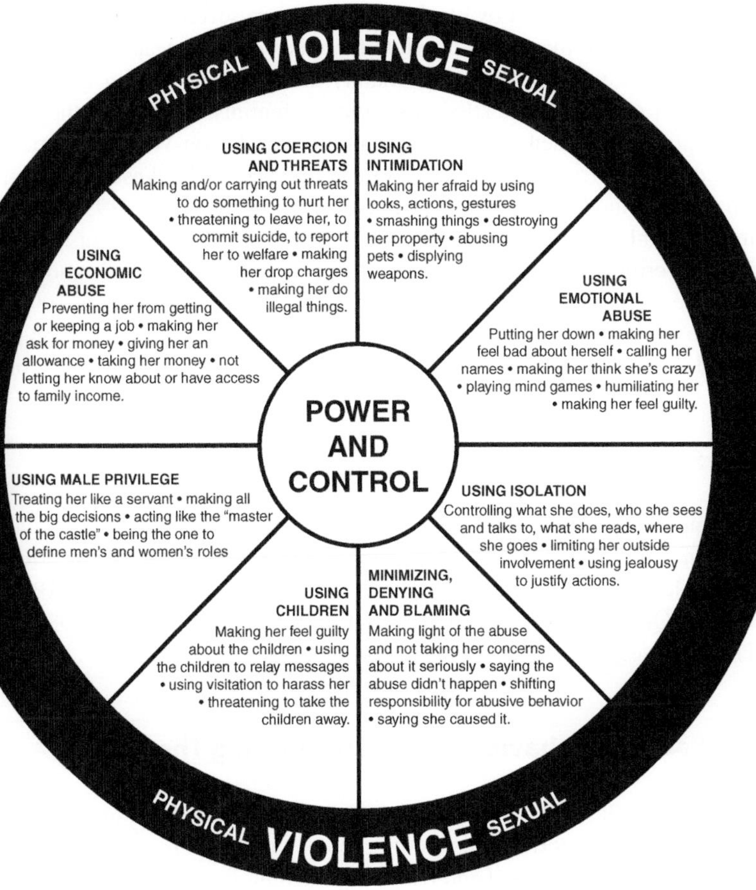

PHYSICAL **VIOLENCE** SEXUAL

USING COERCION AND THREATS
Making and/or carrying out threats to do something to hurt her • threatening to leave her, to commit suicide, to report her to welfare • making her drop charges • making her do illegal things.

USING INTIMIDATION
Making her afraid by using looks, actions, gestures • smashing things • destroying her property • abusing pets • displaying weapons.

USING ECONOMIC ABUSE
Preventing her from getting or keeping a job • making her ask for money • giving her an allowance • taking her money • not letting her know about or have access to family income.

USING EMOTIONAL ABUSE
Putting her down • making her feel bad about herself • calling her names • making her think she's crazy • playing mind games • humiliating her • making her feel guilty.

POWER AND CONTROL

USING MALE PRIVILEGE
Treating her like a servant • making all the big decisions • acting like the "master of the castle" • being the one to define men's and women's roles

USING ISOLATION
Controlling what she does, who she sees and talks to, what she reads, where she goes • limiting her outside involvement • using jealousy to justify actions.

USING CHILDREN
Making her feel guilty about the children • using the children to relay messages • using visitation to harass her • threatening to take the children away.

MINIMIZING, DENYING AND BLAMING
Making light of the abuse and not taking her concerns about it seriously • saying the abuse didn't happen • shifting responsibility for abusive behavior • saying she caused it.

PHYSICAL **VIOLENCE** SEXUAL

Fig. 2.2 The power and control wheel: Duluth model. (Source: Domestic Abuse Intervention Project. Retrieved July 1st, 2019 from https://www.theduluthmodel.org/wheels/)

patriarchal ideology tend to view wife beating not only as acceptable, but also as beneficial and consider women responsible for the violence against them (Carter 2015).

This perspective has been criticised for its stance that DVA can only be perpetrated by men against women. There is some evidence also suggesting that women can be equally as or more violent (Ali and Naylor 2013b; Fiebert 2008). However, this perspective is complex and as a number of commentators including Dobash and Dobash (2004) have highlighted in their own research that DVA is *primarily an asymmetrical problem of men's violence to women, and women's violence does not equate to men's in terms of frequency, severity, consequences and the victim's sense of safety and well-being.*

We would also add that feminism is divided into various forms and some feminists also criticise other feminist perspectives. For instance, black feminists maintain that oppression experienced by black women is more severe and different from that of white women and the voices of white feminists do not speak for the oppression based on racism and classicism that mainly affects black women (Walker 1993). Another form of feminism, called post-colonial feminism, criticises the projection and perception of women from the developing world (non-Western women) as an oppressed, submissive, and voiceless group as opposed to the Western women's projection of being modern, educated, assertive, and powerful (Mills 1998). A group of feminists, mainly from the developing countries (Third world feminism) (Narayan 1997), have criticised Western feminism as being ethnocentric and ignorant of the distinctive experience of women from third world countries (Mohanty 1991). Apart from these types of feminism, there are many other variants or types of the perspective based on geographical location, cultural and religious beliefs, and point of views.

2.1.6   Sociological Perspectives

The sociological perspective of DVA focuses on the social context and situations in which men and women live and where violence takes place. The perspective examines social learning theory, resource theory, exchange theory (Homans 1974), conflict theory (Quinney 1970; Turk 1977), and stress theory (Farrington 1986; Jasinski 2001). In this section, an overview of these theories is presented.

2.2   Learned Behaviour or Social Learning Theory

Social learning (Bandura 1977), also known as "learned behaviour theory", is one of the most popular theories. This theory proposes that both perpetration and acceptance of DVA is a conditioned and learned behaviour. Bandura (1977) believed that the social situation is most important in determining the frequency, form, context in which aggression occurs, and the target of aggressive actions. He argued that men perpetrate abuse because they have seen their fathers being abusive towards their mothers and that women accept abuse because they have seen their mother being abused by their father. This suggests that families play a very important role in not only exposing individuals to the use of violence, but also inculcating an acceptance of the use of violence in relationships. The theory is been used to study the "intergenerational cycle of violence" which proposes that children who witness violence or who have been victims of violence themselves as children are at risk of becoming perpetrators or victims of violence as adults (Black et al. 2010; Cannon et al. 2009; Fehringer and Hindin 2009; Milner et al. 2010). It is also suggested that children who are exposed corporal punishment as a form of disciplining method in childhood learn to consider physical violence as an acceptable method to treat unacceptable behaviour (Afifi et al. 2017). In addition, such children do not learn any other conflict resolution skills.

The studies conducted under this perspective are criticised for the variation of the definition of terms, such as what constitutes witnessing violence as a child and how victimisation and exposure to abuse in childhood is defined? Does this include minor forms of corporal punishment such as mild spanking or does it mean severe punishment (Baumrind et al. 2002; Delsol and Margolin 2004; Gershoff 2002). Besides, findings of studies conducted are inconsistent, as some researchers have identified victimisation as the stronger predictor of DVA than witnessing DVA as a child and others suggest that witnessing DVA as the strongest predictor (Iverson et al. 2011). There is a lack of research investigating the role of these variables in relation to the female perpetrated violence. It is also important to note that not all men who experienced or witnessed abuse as children become perpetrators. Also, not all perpetrators have a history of experiencing or witnessing abuse in childhood.

2.3   Resource Theory

This theory proposed that in an intimate relationship, partner with more resources in terms of income, occupational status, and education may have more say and power in the relationship (Blood and Wolfe 1960). Building on this theory, much research suggests violent intimate or husbands were deficient in resources such as income, education, and occupational status (Atkinson et al. 2005; DeMaris et al. 2003). However, in a meta-analysis, Stith et al. (2004) identified unemployment ($r = -0.10$), lower incomes ($r = -0.08$), and lower education ($r = -0.13$) as weak predictors of male physical violence. In addition, the similar factors (employment: $r = 0.01$; income: $r = -0.04$; education: $r = -0.05$) were reported to have negligible effect sizes and were thus not useful in predicting female victimisation.

Another variant of resource theory is the relevant resource theory which maintains that "it is not so much men's lack of resources that predicts wife abuse, but lack of resources relative to their wives" (Atkinson et al. 2005: 1138). Thus, men who do not enjoy superior status compared with their partners show aggressive and violent behaviour towards them. Various studies have supported this theory and suggest that women with higher incomes or those with unemployed partners are more likely to be abused (Fox et al. 2002; Melzer 2002). Similarly, women with higher educational level (O'Brien 1971) or better occupational status (Atkinson et al. 2005) are more at risk of experiencing DVA.

Resource theory contradicts other theories which suggest that empowering women through education and better employment opportunities is a major strategy to tackle DVA. This perspective is also criticised for not considering gender ideologies and culture and assuming that all men want to be providers for their family (Eirich and Robinson 2017). The application of this theory in societies and cultures that are less patriarchal in nature is questioned. On the other hand, men in patriarchal societies are more resourceful and are considered superior, though violence still exists.

2.3.1   Nested Ecological Framework Theory

The nested ecological framework is one of the most widely used accounts of DVA (Bronfenbrenner 1977, 1979, 1986). The framework offers a comprehensive view of

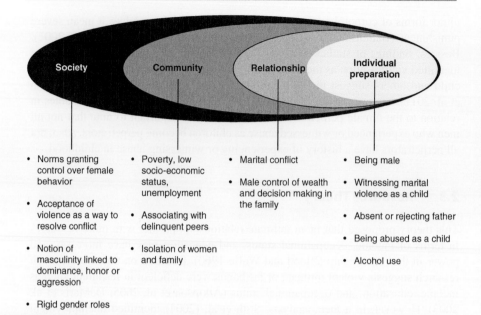

Fig. 2.3 Ecological model of factors associated with partner abuse (Source: Heise, L. L. (1998). Violence against women: An integrated, ecological framework. *Violence Against Women, 4,* 262-290)

the issue of DVA by looking at different factors at various levels. The model suggests that behaviours are influenced by interaction at various levels of social organisation (Ali and Naylor 2013b). The framework has four levels: individual; relational; community; and societal (see Fig. 2.3). The individual level covers the biological and personal factors (age, gender, education, income, psychological problems, personality disorders, aggressive tendencies, and substance abuse) which influence individual behaviour. The next level known as relations encompasses the family, including intimate partner, friends, and workplace situations. The next level related to the role of community where the person lives, develops relationships and interacts with friends, school-mates, and work colleagues. The final level of the framework is the societal level that relates to the structures and systems of the society and culture where the person lives. It also looks at the factors, including parental role and responsibilities, societal norms, larger economic, social and health structures affecting peoples' lives. The model also suggests that to deal with DVA, it is the interaction of various factors at different levels that needs to be understood.

2.4   Biological Explanations

The biological or organic explanations of DVA explore genetic, congenital, and organic causes of behaviour resulting from genetic defects, head injury, and hormonal and chemical anomalies.

2.4.1   Genetics

There have been some attempts to explore links between genetics and abusive behaviour. Hines and colleague (Hines and Saudino 2002) explored the relationship between genetic and environmental factors and individual differences in intimate aggression (Hines and Saudino 2002: 701). Findings revealed familial resemblance in psychological and physical DVA attributable to shared genes. Genetic influence could explain 16% and 15% of the variance in the use and receipt of physical aggression, respectively. Likewise, 22% and 25% of the variance in the use and receipt of psychological aggression was attributable to genetic factors (Hines and Saudino 2004). In another study, Saudino and Hines (2007) suggested a genetic influence on victims of violence or aggression due to evocative or active genotype environment correlation. Evocative correlation refers to the victim's genetically influenced behaviours that could induce aggressive reaction from others. The active genotype environment correlation, however, refers to victim's tendency to select aggressive partners due to a congruence between genetically influenced traits. Research suggests that aggression and the ability to control aggression are genetically influenced and some people may act more aggressively than others and that genetic factors coupled with environmental influences increase the risk of aggressive, antisocial, and criminal behaviour (Barnes et al. 2013; Stuart et al. 2014). Much research is needed to explore genetic influences on abusive behaviour and to further understand the relationship between biological factors and DVA.

2.4.2   Head Injury

Head injury is identified as one of the precursors of aggressive behaviour. Head injury not only affects the survivor, but it also affects their family members and friends. The long-term impacts of head injury include changes in survivor's personality, irritability, rage outbursts, and reduced impulse control (Wood et al. 2005). Personality changes resulting from head injury may also have an impact on the quality of intimate relationship contributing to conflicts and DVA. However, we know that no all violent men have sustained head injuries and not everyone with a history of head injury is abusive to their partner.

2.4.3   Neurotransmitters

Attempts have been made to explore the association between DVA and various neurotransmitters (serotonin, dopamine, gamma-aminobutyric acid (GABA), glutamate, and norepinephrine, substance P, acetylcholine, vasopressin, oxytocin, testosterone, and cortisol). Among these, a positive association between testosterone and aggression has already been established in animals, but remains under-investigated and inconclusive in humans (Corvo and Dutton 2015). At the same time, a lower level of serotonin is identified as predictive of impulsive and violent behaviour. Decreased serotonin levels have a negative effect on mood and behaviour, whereas increased serotonin levels result in improved social interaction and decreased aggression (Corvo and Dutton 2015).

2.5 Psychological Explanations

The psychological explanations focus on factors affecting the individual perpetrator or the victim-survivor. The role of various psychological and psychiatric problems including psychopathology, personality disorders, attachment needs, anger/hostility, substance and alcohol abuse, self-esteem, and individual abilities (assertiveness, communication, problem-solving skills) are explored.

2.5.1 Psychopathology and Personality Theories

The initial theories exploring DVA were based on the psychopathological orientation of violence. Arising from the findings of studies conducted on known violent men in prisons, community-based settings or victim women in shelters, it was hypothesised that men who perpetrate violence and women who experience violence suffer from mental health problems such as depression, borderline personality organisation and psychopathology and antisocial personality (Chester and DeWall 2018). Antisocial perpetrators use DVA with or without provocation, whereas those with borderline personality disorder perpetrate DVA reactively. We also know that women victims of DVA suffer from borderline personality symptomology (BPS), depressive disorders, anxiety, posttraumatic stress disorder, psychological distress, substance dependence, or suicidality. Evidence also suggests that people with psychiatric disorders regardless of gender are prone to get involved in abusive relationships (Ehrensaft et al. 2006).

Research in this area has been conducted on either prisoners, court referred cases, people attending treatment programmes, or women in shelters and therefore, the findings of such studies have limited generalisability. In addition, not everyone with psychopathology reacts violently towards their intimates; and not every violent person has a psychopathological disorder. Opponents also believe that considering psychopathology as the sole cause of violence distracts society from examining and dealing with other factors such as societal attitudes, cultural norms, and structural inequalities that condone violence.

2.5.2 Attachment Theory

Attachment theory proposes that DVA could be a result of disturbed attachment to ones' partner (Bowlby 1988). Attachment is a process by which an infant seeks closeness to mother (or her substitute) specifically in perceived distressing situations. An infant attaches to an adult who remains a constant caregiver in the initial

6–24 months of their life and who respond sensitively to the infant in social interactions. Bowlby believed that trust in the attachment figure and an assurance about the availability and accessibility of the attachment figure or vice versa develops slowly during infancy and continues to build in childhood and adolescence in its various forms. Expectations developed during initial days of life remain relatively unchanged throughout life (Bowlby 1973: 235). These expectations and the response of the attachment figure to the expectations lead to the development of "internal working models" that direct the individual's feelings, beliefs, and expectations in later relationships. Bowlby maintained that disturbed or unmet attachment needs result in the development and provocation of interpersonal anger, and a feeling of rage. A perceived threat of separation or loss of an attachment figure generates feelings of terror, grief, and rage in the infant (Bowlby 1969, 1973). Repeated experiences of unmet attachment needs during childhood may lead to the development of disturbed attachment patterns in adult relationships. This theory was applied to adult relationship and Hazan and Shaver (1987) proposed romantic love as an attachment process and developed an instrument to measure the adult version of the infantile attachment patterns (secure, ambivalent, and anxious-avoidant). Further studies confirmed the similarity between attachment patterns of children–adults and romantic and intimate relationship in adult life (Sutton 2019). Research related to attachment theory can help identify people at risk of becoming abusive; understand why they act in that way; which behaviours to expect; what circumstances force them to behave in that manner; and what could be the consequences (Gormley 2005). Attachment theory, however, does not explain the role of biological factors or why children from one family do not all behave the same (Ali and Naylor 2013a).

2.5.3 Anger/Hostility

Work has been undertaken to explore link between anger/hostility and DVA. Evidence suggests that violent partners experience more anger and hostility towards their partner than non-violent partners (Baron et al. 2007; Norlander and Eckhardt 2005). A critical examination of the literature points out that findings about the relationship between anger, hostility, and DVA are inconsistent (Ali and Naylor 2013a). While we know that anger contributes to DVA, the concept of anger remains poorly defined and underexplored. The difference between anger and hostility is not clear. In addition, considering anger as the cause of DVA partly blames the victim for arousing anger and therefore requires them to change their behaviour to reduce abuse. It also helps abusers use anger as an excuse of their behaviour and consequently to deny the responsibility of their behaviour.

2.5.4 Self-Esteem

Low self-esteem is identified as another psychological factor contributing to DVA, though research findings in this regard are inconsistent. It is suggested that violent partners suffer from low self-esteem and use DVA in an attempt to defend or cover up their feelings of inferiority and shame and to improve their own feeling of self-worth (Papadakaki et al. 2009).

2.6 Communication Skills and Assertiveness

Evidence suggests that violent men tend to suffer from poor communication skills and display aversive behaviour (Babcock et al. 2011; Waltz et al. 2000), are offensive and negative, or defensive and negative, and engage in less positive or constructive communication (Berns et al. 1999; Holtzworth-Munroe et al. 1998) when interacting with their partner, compared with non-violent men. It has been suggested that violent partners tend to lack these skills and use violence when they are unable to resolve conflicts (Ramos Salazar 2015). Researchers have investigated two types of assertiveness including general assertiveness (being able to behave assertive generally in any situation) and spouse-specific assertiveness (an ability to behave assertively with one's spouse). However, the results of these studies are not consistent, as some report a lack of spouse specific assertiveness only and others report a lack of spouse-specific assertiveness and general assertiveness abilities or a lack of general assertiveness abilities only (Satyanarayana et al. 2015).

2.6.1 Substance and Alcohol Abuse

Alcohol use and abuse remain significantly associated with DVA (Choenni et al. 2017). Research in this area can be categorised into three groups; studies supporting an association between alcohol or substance abuse and DVA perpetration; studies supporting an association between alcohol or substance abuse and victimisation; and studies that identify a reciprocal relationship between alcohol abuse and both perpetration and victimisation (Stith et al. 2004; Thompson and Kingree 2006). In addition, violence perpetrated by alcoholic men was more frequent and severe than that perpetrated by non-alcoholic men (Choenni et al. 2017). Women's perpetration of DVA as well as women's victimisation of DVA reported to have an association with substance or alcohol abuse (Parks and Fals-Stewart 2004). Victims also use or abuse alcohol and or substance as a coping strategy (Simmons et al. 2008). Though it is difficult to establish a causal link between alcohol and substance abuse and DVA, these are important contributing factors. The opponent of this perspective maintains that endorsing such association means taking away the responsibility from men and providing them with an excuse for justifying their violence. This account remains an avenue for further research (Testa and Derrick 2014; Testa et al. 2012).

Available evidence suggests that psychopathology, personality disorders, attachment needs, anger/hostility, substance and alcohol abuse, self-esteem, and individual abilities such as assertiveness, communication and problem-solving skills can help understand DVA to some extent. Opponents of each of these explanations have questioned why not all men behave the same? It is important to note here that none of the factors is identified as the sole cause, as the findings of the studies remain inconsistent and further research is warranted with regard to all psychological explanations.

Time to Reflect
In this chapter, we have presented an overview of a number of theories and explanations for DVA. Please take a moment to consider the following:

- **What theory or perspective did you find most interesting and why?—What questions did this raise for you?**
- **What theory or perspective did you find most challenging and why?—What questions did this raise for you?**
- **Consider what further reading and exploration you need to undertake in order to answer your questions.**

2.7   Summary

This chapter has explored various explanations of DVA. It appears that factors like the ideology of patriarchy, culture and society, religion, media, and individual characteristics come together to explain DVA. Biological perspective sees the issue of DVA as being secondary to aggression, which results from structural and chemical changes in the brain due, for example, to trauma or head injury. Psychopathological theories consider that DVA results from psychopathology, mental illness, inability to anger and hostility, attachment problems, deficiency in various skills and abilities such as management of anger and hostility, lack of assertiveness, self-esteem, and communication skills. The feminist perspective blames men, patriarchal structure of the societies, power and control issues, and learned helplessness. The sociological perspective assumes violence in the family of origin, differences in the possession of resources of men and women, conflict in the family, and stress as the explanatory factors. Finally, the nested ecological framework looks at various factors at various levels in the family, community, and society to explain the phenomenon of violence in intimate relationships. The review makes it clear that no single theory or factor can fully explain DVA, but every perspective contributes to the explanation and provides an important insight into the issue of abuse. Each also has its limitations, so in understanding DVA, it may be useful to draw on multiple explanations.

Summary Points
- There are various explanations of DVA proposed.
- Each explanation has been critiqued for what it has to offer in understanding DVA.
- It may be helpful to conceptualise DVA as having multiple explanations.

Web Resource

https://www.who.int/violenceprevention/approach/ecology/en/

References

Afifi TO, Mota N, Sareen J, MacMillan HL (2017) The relationships between harsh physical punishment and child maltreatment in childhood and intimate partner violence in adulthood. BMC Public Health 17(1):493

Ali PA, Naylor PB (2013a) Intimate partner violence: a narrative review of the biological and psychological explanations for its causation. Aggress Violent Behav 18(3):373–382

Ali PA, Naylor PB (2013b) Intimate partner violence: a narrative review of the feminist, social and ecological explanations for its causation. Aggress Violent Behav 18(6):611–619

Atkinson MP, Greenstein TN, Lang MM (2005) For women, breadwinning can be dangerous: gendered resource theory and wife abuse. J Marriage Fam 67:1137–1148

Babcock JC, Graham K, Canady B, Ross JM (2011) A proximal change experiment testing two communication exercises with intimate partner violent men. Behav Ther 42(2):336–347. https://doi.org/10.1016/j.beth.2010.08.010

Ball P, Wyman E (1978) Battered wives and powerlessness: what can counselors do? Victimology 2:545–557

Bandura A (1977) Social learning theory. General Learning Press, New York

Barnes JC, TenEyck M, Boutwell BB, Beaver KM (2013) Indicators of domestic/intimate partner violence are structured by genetic and nonshared environmental influences. J Psychiatr Res 47(3):371–376

Baron K, Smith T, Butner J, Nealey-Moore J, Hawkins M, Uchino B (2007) Hostility, anger, and marital adjustment: concurrent and prospective associations with psychosocial vulnerability. J Behav Med 30(1):1–10

Baumrind D, Lazerle RE, Cowan PA (2002) Ordinary physical punishment: is it harmful? Comment on Gershoff. Psychol Bull 128:580–589

Berns SB, Jacobson NS, Gottman JM (1999) Demand/withdraw interaction patterns between different types of batterers and their spouses. J Marital Fam Ther 25(3):337–348

Bhandari M, Sprague S, Tornetta P 3rd, D'Aurora V, Schemitsch E, Shearer H et al (2008) (Mis) perceptions about intimate partner violence in women presenting for orthopaedic care: a survey of Canadian orthopaedic surgeons. J Bone Joint Surg Am 90(7):1590–1597

Black DS, Sussman S, Unger JB (2010) A further look at the intergenerational transmission of violence: witnessing interparental violence in emerging adulthood. J Interpers Violence 25(6):1022–1042

Blood RO, Wolfe DM (1960) Husbands and wives. Free Press, Glencoe

Bowlby J (1969) Attachment and loss: Vol I. Attachment. Basic Books, New York

Bowlby J (1973) Attachment and loss: Vol II. Separation. Basic Books, New York

Bowlby J (1988) A secure base: parent child attachment and healthy human development. Basic Books, New York

Bronfenbrenner U (1977) Toward an experimental ecology of human development. Am Psychol 32(7):513–531

Bronfenbrenner U (1979) The ecology of human development: experiments by nature and design. Harvard University Press, Cambridge

Bronfenbrenner U (1986) Ecology of the family as a context for human development: research perspectives. Dev Psychol 22(6):723–742

Cannon EA, Bonomi AE, Anderson ML, Rivara FP (2009) The intergenerational transmission of witnessing intimate partner violence. Arch Pediatr Adolesc Med 163(8):706–708

Carter J (2015) Patriarchy and violence against women and girls. Lancet 385(9978):e40–e41

Chester DS, DeWall CN (2018) The roots of intimate partner violence. Curr Opin Psychol 19:55–59. https://doi.org/10.1016/j.copsyc.2017.04.009

Choenni V, Hammink A, van de Mheen D (2017) Association between substance use and the perpetration of family violence in industrialized countries: a systematic review. Trauma Violence Abuse 18(1):37–50. https://doi.org/10.1177/1524838015589253

Corvo K, Dutton D (2015) Neurotransmitter and neurochemical factors in domestic violence perpetration: implications for theory development. Partn Abus 6(3):351–364

Craven Z (2003) Battered woman syndrome. Australian domestic and family violence clearinghouse. http://www.austdvclearinghouse.unsw.edu.au/PDF%20files/battered%20_woman_syndrome.pdf

Delsol C, Margolin G (2004) The role of family-of-origin violence in men's marital violence perpetration. Clin Psychol Rev 24(1):99–122

DeMaris A, Benson ML, Fox GL, Hill T, Wyk JV (2003) Distal and proximal factors in domestic violence: a test of an integrated model. J Marriage Fam 65:652–667

Dobash RP, Dobash RE (2004) Women's violence to men in intimate relationships: working on a puzzle. Br J Criminol 44(3):324–349

Ehrensaft MK, Moffitt TE, Caspi A (2006) Is domestic violence followed by an increased risk of psychiatric disorders among women but not among men? A longitudinal cohort study. Am J Psychiatry 163(5):885–892. https://doi.org/10.1176/appi.ajp.163.5.885

Eirich GM, Robinson JH (2017) Does earning more than your spouse increase your financial satisfaction? A comparison of men and women in the United States, 1982 to 2012. J Fam Issues 38(17):2371–2399

Farrington K (1986) The application of stress theory to the study of family violence: principles, problems and prospects. J Fam Violence 1:131–149

Fehringer JA, Hindin MJ (2009) Like parent, like child: intergenerational transmission of partner violence in Cebu, the Philippines. J Adolesc Health 44(4):363–371

Fiebert MS (2008) References examining assaults by women on their spouses or male partners: an annotated bibliography. http://www.csulb.edu/~mfiebert/assault.htm

Fox GL, Benson ML, DeMaris AA, Wyk JV (2002) Economic distress and intimate violence: testing family stress and resources theories. J Marriage Fam 64(3):793–807

García-Moreno C, Jansen HAFM, Ellsberg M, Heise L, Watts C (2005) WHO multi-country study on women's health and domestic violence against women: initial results onprevalence, health outcomes and women's responses. World Health Organization, Geneva

Gershoff ET (2002) Corporal punishment by parents and associated child behaviors and experiences: a meta-analytic and theoretical review. Psychol Bull 128(4):539–579

Gormley B (2005) An adult attachment theoretical perspective of gender symmetry in intimate partner violence. Sex Roles 52:785–795

Haj-Yahia MM, Schiff M (2007) Definitions of and beliefs about wife abuse among undergraduate students of social work. Int J Offender Ther Comp Criminol 51(2):170–190. https://doi.org/10.1177/0306624x06291457

Hazan C, Shaver P (1987) Romantic love conceptualized as an attachment process. J Pers Soc Psychol 52(3):511–524

Hines DA, Saudino KJ (2002) Intergenerational transmission of intimate partner violence. Trauma Violence Abuse 3:210–225. https://doi.org/10.1177/15248380020033004

Hines DA, Saudino KJ (2004) Genetic and environmental influences on intimate partner aggression: a preliminary study. Violence Vict 19:701–718

Holtzworth-Munroe A, Smutzler N, Stuart GL (1998) Demand and withdraw communication among couples experiencing husband violence. J Consult Clin Psychol 66(5):731–743

Homans GC (1974) Social behavior; its elementary forms (Revised ed.). Harcourt, Brace, Jovanovich, New York

Iverson KM, Jimenez S, Harrington KM, Resick PA (2011) The contribution of childhood family violence on later intimate partner violence among robbery victims. Violence Vict 26(1):73–87

Jasinski JL (2001) Theoretical explanations for violence against women. In: Renzetti CM, Edleson JL, Bergen RK (eds) The sourcebook on violence against women. Sage Publications, Thousand Oaks, pp 5–22

McPhail BA, Busch NB, Kulkarni S, Rice S (2007) An integrative feminist model: the evolving feminist perspective on intimate partner violence. Violence Against Women 13:817–841

Melzer SA (2002) Gender, work, and intimate violence: men's occupational violence spillover and compensatory violence. J Marriage Fam 64(4):820–832

Mills S (1998) Postcolonial feminist theory. In: Jackson S, Jones J (eds) Contemporary feminist theories. Edinburgh University Press, Edinburgh

Milner JS, Thomsen CJ, Crouch JL, Rabenhorst MM, Martens PM, Dyslin CW et al (2010) Do trauma symptoms mediate the relationship between childhood physical abuse and adult child abuse risk? Child Abuse Negl 34(5):332–344

Mohanty CT (1991) Introduction. In: Mohanty CT, Russo A, Torres L (eds) In third world women and the politics of feminism. Indiana University Press, Bloomington

Mossière A, Maeder EM, Pica E (2018) Racial composition of couples in battered spouse syndrome cases: a look at juror perceptions and decisions. J Interpers Violence 33(18):2867–2890. https://doi.org/10.1177/0886260516632355

Narayan U (1997) Dislocating cultures: identities, traditions, and third-world feminism. Routledge, New York

Naved R, Azim S, Bhuiya A, Persson L (2006) Physical violence by husbands: magnitude, disclosure and help seeking behaviour of women in Bangladesh. Soc Sci Med 62:2917–2929

Norlander B, Eckhardt C (2005) Anger, hostility, and male perpetrators of intimate partner violence: a meta-analytic review. Clin Psychol Rev 25(2):119–152

O'Brien JE (1971) Violence in divorce prone families. J Marriage Fam 33(4):692–698.

Overmier JB, Seligman MEP (1967) Effects of inescapable shock upon subsequent escape and avoidance responding. J Comp Physiol Psychol 63:28–33

Papadakaki M, Tzamalouka GS, Chatzifotiou S, Chliaoutakis J (2009) Seeking for risk factors of intimate partner violence (IPV) in a Greek National Sample. J Interpers Violence:732–750. https://doi.org/10.1177/0886260508317181

Parks KA, Fals-Stewart W (2004) The temporal relationship between college women's alcohol consumption and victimization experiences. Alcohol Clin Exp Res 28:625–629

Pease B (2000) Recreating men: post modern masculinity politics. Sage, London

Quinney R (1970) The social reality of crime. Little Brown, Boston

Ramos Salazar L (2015) The negative reciprocity process in marital relationships: a literature review. Aggress Violent Behav 24:113–119. https://doi.org/10.1016/j.avb.2015.05.008

Satyanarayana VA, Hebbani S, Hegde S, Krishnan S, Srinivasan K (2015) Two sides of a coin: perpetrators and survivors perspectives on the triad of alcohol, intimate partner violence and mental health in South India. Asian J Psychiatr 15:38–43. https://doi.org/10.1016/j.ajp.2015.04.014

Saudino K, Hines D (2007) Etiological similarities between psychological and physical aggression in intimate relationships: a behavioral genetic exploration. J Fam Violence 22(3):121–129

Seligman ME, Maier SF (1967) Failure to escape traumatic shock. J Exp Psychol 74:1–9

Simmons CA, Lehmann P, Cobb N (2008) Women arrested for partner violence and substance use: an exploration of discrepancies in the literature. J Interpers Violence 23:707–727

Stith SM, Smith DB, Penn CE, Ward DB, Tritt D (2004) Intimate partner physical abuse perpetration and victimization risk factors: a meta-analytic review. Aggress Violent Behav 10(1):65–98

Stuart GL, McGeary JE, Shorey RC, Knopik VS, Beaucage K, Temple JR (2014) Genetic associations with intimate partner violence in a sample of hazardous drinking men in batterer intervention programs. Violence Against Women 20(4):385–400

Sutton TE (2019) Review of attachment theory: familial predictors, continuity and change, and intrapersonal and relational outcomes. Marriage Fam Rev 55(1):1–22. https://doi.org/10.1080/01494929.2018.1458001

Testa M, Derrick JL (2014) A daily process examination of the temporal association between alcohol use and verbal and physical aggression in community couples. Psychol Addict Behav 28(1):127

Testa M, Kubiak A, Quigley BM, Houston RJ, Derrick JL, Levitt A et al (2012) Husband and wife alcohol use as independent or interactive predictors of intimate partner violence. J Stud Alcohol Drugs 73(2):268–276. https://doi.org/10.15288/jsad.2012.73.268

Thompson MP, Kingree JB (2006) The roles of victim and perpetrator alcohol use in intimate partner violence outcomes. J Interpers Violence 21:163–177. https://doi.org/10.1177/0886260505282283

Turk A (1977) Class, conflict, and criminalization. Sociol Focus 10:209–220

Waites EA (1978) Female masochism and the enforced restriction of choice. Victimology 2:535–544

Walker L (1977/1978) Battered women and learned helplessness. Victimology 2:525–534

Walker L (1979) The battered woman. Harper & Row, New York

Walker A (1993) In search of our mothers' gardens: Womanist prose. Harcourt Brace Jovanovich, San Diego

Walker LA (2006) Battered woman syndrome: empirical findings. Ann N Y Acad Sci 1087:142–157

Walker L, Browne A (1985) Gender and victimization by intimates. J Pers 53:179–195

Waltz J, Babcock JC, Jacobson NS, Gottman JM (2000) Testing a typology of batterers. J Consult Clin Psychol 68(4):658

Wood RL, Liossi C, Wood L (2005) The impact of head injury neurobehavioural sequelae on personal relationships: preliminary findings. Brain Inj 19(10):845–851

Classifications of Domestic Violence and Abuse

3

Parveen Ali and Julie McGarry

3.1 Introduction

The role of healthcare professionals in recognizing and responding to DVA cannot be underestimated. While healthcare professionals often understand the manifestations and health impacts of DVA, they do not always understand the theoretical underpinning of the concept of DVA. Over the past few decades, researchers have tried to explain DVA through various classifications. Some are based on the forms of abuse; others are on perpetrator's attributes, whereas some are based on a combination of these approaches. This chapter aims to present a number of classifications of DVA. We use the word 'typology' and 'classification' interchangeably and only commonly reported typologies are presented. Forms of abuse, such as physical, psychological, sexual and financial abuse and coercive control, is identified as one typology; however, we have already explored these in Chap. 1, so let's look at other typologies in this chapter.

You may think why do we need to know about classifications? Well, knowing about various classifications or typologies can help us understand the complexities of DVA, various causes, correlates, and consequences. Perpetrators and their victims (or survivors) are not a homogenous group of individuals, but those with a

P. Ali (✉)
School of Health Sciences, The University of Sheffield, Sheffield, UK
e-mail: parveen.ali@sheffield.ac.uk

J. McGarry
School of Health Sciences, The University of Nottingham, Queen's Medical Centre, Nottingham, UK
e-mail: Julie.McGarry@nottingham.ac.uk; https://institutemh.org.uk/research/centre-for-social-futures/projects/349-research-area-domestic-violence-and-abuse

© Springer Nature Switzerland AG 2020
P. Ali, J. McGarry (eds.), *Domestic Violence in Health Contexts: A Guide for Healthcare Professions*, https://doi.org/10.1007/978-3-030-29361-1_3

multitude of individual and compound precipitating and exacerbating factors affecting their circumstances and thereby behaviour. Knowing about classifications may also help develop appropriate empirical assessments, targeted interventions, ways through which such interventions and preventive approaches can be measured effectively. It may also help in developing appropriate and accurate screening instruments to assess the risk of DVA in health and social care settings. Such differentiation may also help develop family-law decisions about post-separation parenting (i.e. appropriateness of parent–child contact; safeguarding requirements; and parenting plans are likely to promote healthy outcomes for children and parent–child relationships), by considering the type of DVA and its effect on the victim-parent and the children.

3.2 Types of Domestic Violence and Abuse

In the following, two common typologies explained by Johnson (1995) and Johnston and Campbell (1993) are explained.

3.2.1 Johnson's Typology

Michael Johnson, an American sociologist, developed and, over time, refined his proposed typology (Johnson 1995, 2008; Kelly and Johnson 2008). His work has been most influential of the typologies presented so far. Johnson (1995) initially proposed two forms of DVA known as 'patriarchal terrorism' and 'common couple violence'. Though, following further expansion and development, the typology now consists of five types and these are: Coercive Controlling Violence (CCV), Violent Resistance, Situational Couple Violence (SCV), Mutual Violent Control Violence, and Separation-Instigated Violence.

3.2.1.1 Coercive Controlling Violence (CCV)
CCV denotes to a pattern of emotionally abusive behaviours characterized of intimidation, coercion, and control together with physical abuse in an intimate relationship (Kelly and Johnson 2008: 478). It refers to a pattern of control and manipulation by one partner against the other and how the coercive partner keeps the victim under scrutiny and sets the rules in the relationship. Failure to follow such rules often results in punitive action against the victim (Beck et al. 2013; Tanha et al. 2010). The abuser uses one or more tactics such as intimidation, emotional abuse, isolation, minimizing, denying, and blaming, use of children, asserting male privilege, economic abuse, coercion, and threats to keep the victim in their control. This type of abuse was first described as 'Patriarchal Terrorism' followed by 'Intimate Terrorism', and is now known as CCV. This type of abuse is more severe, escalates over time and occurs more frequently. In heterosexual relationships, CCV is most often perpetrated by men (Ansara and Hindin 2010; Ansara and Hindin 2011; Gulliver and Fanslow 2015), though there is some evidence suggesting that women can also be

CCV perpetrators in both heterosexual and same-sex relationships (Beck et al. 2013; Hines et al. 2007; Eckstein 2017).

3.2.1.2 Violent Resistance

This type of violence is used by the victim of violence to resist violence from a coercive controlling partner. Other terms used to describe this type of violence include Female Resistance, Resistive/Reactive Violence, Self-Defence (Beck et al. 2013; Kelly and Johnson 2008), and battered women syndrome (Walker 1984; Yllö and Bograd 1988). Johnson explained that a man or woman can resort to violence in an attempt to stop the violence or to stand up for themselves. For many women, use of self-protective violence may be almost automatic and happens as soon as the perpetrator begins to use violence. However, most women find out quickly that responding with violence is ineffective and may, in fact, worsen the situation and they may end up sustaining more and severe injuries. While much research has been conducted to explore the violent resistive behaviour of women who murdered their intimate partners, research on men's resistive behaviour is still scarce.

3.2.1.3 Situational Couple Violence (SCV)

This refers to the type of violence between partners when an individual can be violent and non-controlling in a relationship with a non-violent partner or a violent but non-controlling partner (Johnson 2006). It is the most common type of violence in the general population and can be perpetrated by male or female. This type of abuse stems from situations, arguments, and conflicts between partners, which then escalate into physical abuse (Kelly and Johnson 2008). Such abuse results from one or both partner's inability to manage conflict or anger. The frequency and intensity of violence doesn't increase over time and usually involves minor forms of violence compared with CCV. SCV may consist of verbally abusive acts such as cursing, shouting, name calling, and accusations of infidelity. Unlike CCV, it does not have a chronic pattern of controlling, intimidating, and stalking behaviours (Kelly and Johnson 2008). Other terms used to describe this type include Common Couple Violence, Male-Controlling Interactive Violence, and Conflict Motivated Violence (Ellis and Stuckless 1996, 2006).

3.2.1.4 Mutual Violent Control Violence

This type of violence occurs when both partners are violent and controlling, also known as two intimate terrorists (Beck et al. 2013). It is a rare type of violence and not much is known about its features, frequency, and consequences (Johnson 2000; Johnson and Ferraro 2000; Kelly and Johnson 2008).

3.2.1.5 Separation-Instigated Violence

This type of violence occurs in couples who are in the process of separation and divorce (McKay et al. 2018). Such couples do not normally have a history of DVA in their relationship and the violent episodes are triggered in response to traumatic experiences at the time of separation. Such experiences include finding the home empty after the spouse's (and perhaps, children's) departure, humiliation, and insult faced as a result of separation and divorce (especially if the person is a known figure), and allegations of sexual abuse. The violence in such situation represents an atypical and serious loss of psychological control. Such violence is typically limited to one or two mild to more severe forms of violent episodes during the separation period (Kelly and Johnson 2008: 487). Seen symmetrically in both men and women, this type of violence is more likely to be perpetrated by the spouse who is left and/ or is shocked by divorce action and feel rejected. The various ways a person may react include lashing out, throwing objects at the spouse, destroying property, and trying to intimidate the spouse or her new partner through various acts including sideswiping (to strike along the side in passing) or damaging their car (Kelly and Johnson 2008).

To sum up, the focus of this classification is not the seriousness or frequency of violence, but in the presence or absence of control (Johnson and Leone 2005), though physical abuse is prevalent in all five types.

3.2.2 Johnston's Typology

Another typology is proposed by Janet Johnston and colleagues who attempted to differentiate between types of DVA in the context of child custody and access disputes (Johnston and Campbell 1993) by studying divorcing parents. They proposed five types of DVA and these included ongoing and episodic male battering, female initiated violence, separation-engendered violence, male-controlling interactive violence, and violence due to psychotic and paranoid reactions (Johnston and Campbell 1993).

3.2.2.1 Episodic Male Battering
This type of violence is initiated by men against their partner and may be present in up to 18% of high-conflict divorcing families (Johnston and Campbell 1993). It is similar to CCV identified by Johnson (Kelly and Johnson 2008). Female initiated violence may be present in 15% of high-conflict divorcing families. Moderately severe violence can occur if the perpetrator loses control while restraining the attacking partner (Johnston and Campbell 1993).

3.2.2.2 Separation-Engendered Violence
This type of violence occurs only during or after the separation and usually there is no violence during the marriage or relationship itself. This type of violence can be present in up to 25% of high-conflict divorcing families. The physical violence is generally initiated by the partner—male or female—who feels rejected. This is similar to Kelly and Johnson's (2008) separation-instigated violence.

3.2.2.3 Male-Controlling Interactive Violence
This type of violence arises from mutual verbal arguments and insults progressing to physical violence. It happens in up to 20% of high-conflict divorcing families. Violence can be initiated by either partner; however, the man may physically

dominate or overpower the woman. In addition, a woman's struggles and counterattacks may result in man becoming more dangerous and threatening (Johnston and Campbell 1993). This type of violence is similar to SCV (Kelly and Johnson 2008).

3.2.2.4 Psychotic and Paranoid Reactions

This type of violence is present in up to 65% of high-conflict divorcing families (Johnston and Campbell 1993) though more evidence is needed to understand this type.

Case Study 1: Love

The following case study is a real-life account; however, names and details are changed.

Ela was a successful physician, married to Adam, a successful surgeon. To the outside world they appeared to be professionally successful and in a happy relationship. They were together for 13 years and had two children under the age of 12. Ela was recalled as being a confident person with a good sense of humour and an outgoing personality, whereas Adam appeared to be a shy, reserved, and withdrawn and did not really like to be in social gatherings.

Tensions in their life started in the first year of living together. In public, they looked like an ideal, loving couple. In private, however, Adam was verbally abusive, would ridicule Ela, mock and criticize her appearance, for example, drawing attention to her weight. He would not eat the food that Ela cooked for him and was not interested in supporting Ela either professionally or personally. Adam had also been physically abusive on several occasions and was reported to police. Although, he always managed to persuade Ela to reconcile and withdraw her complaints, thus enabling withdrawal of criminal charges.

Ela's family and friend were baffled as to why Ela wanted to stay in such a relationship. She was educated, financially independent, and surrounded by a devoted support network. Some friends believed that she loved Adam and that she was an optimist who believed that things would change in her relationship. Their relationship was imbalanced in many ways with Ela having responsibility for most household tasks. Ela would always be checking in with Adam, seeking his permission before making decisions. When she was out with other people, Adam would call repeatedly, demanding to know who she was with and what she was doing. Adam also totally controlled her social media presence: he persuaded her to 'unfriend' people he didn't approve of and post only the photos he selected. He was also in control at home. She needed to ask his permission for everything. He forbade her to let their children play with children who didn't live up to his standards. He criticized her parenting, saying that she needed to do more and do better. He called her stupid and useless and used language such as 'I should have left you', or 'I would have been better off without you'. However, outside the home and in his professional life, Adam had a good reputation.

Tensions grew and the episodes of violence and abuse escalated. Ela started thinking and talking about separation and divorce. Adam panicked and begged her for time to 'do we have a quote'. Ela suspected that Adam had an affair. Over the next few months, Ela thoughts about divorce firmed. She began an affair with a fellow colleague and involved a lawyer whom she shared her experiences of an abusive marriage. She told the lawyer that she could no longer tolerate the violence in her household. If her children had been one of the reasons why she wanted to make her marriage work before, now, she decided, she needed to get out for their sake. Her lawyer wrote to Adam telling him about Ela's intention to divorce him. Ela moved into the basement of the house, but Adam kept taking her things back up into their bedroom. Shortly afterwards Ela was nowhere to be found in the house. When asked, Adam told Ela's family that she had left in the night with a suitcase and her boyfriend. Two days later, Ela's body was found in the same suitcase beside a river. She had died of manual asphyxiation and blunt force trauma causing injuries all over her body, including a broken neck and broken ribs.

Time to Reflect
You have explored various classifications in this chapter. In this activity, we would like you to examine this case study in relation to various classifications presented. See if all classifications can be applied to this case study?

3.3   Typology by Perpetrator: Men

Perpetrator or batterer refers to the abuser of violence and a few classifications are offered to classify perpetrators based on their presenting characteristics. The common typologies include typology by Holtzworth-Munroe and typology by Jacobson and Gottman, and these are described below.

3.3.1   Holtzworth-Munroe's Typology

Holtzworth-Munroe and Stuart (1994) reviewed 15 previous perpetrator typologies to propose theirs. The authors (1994) offered three subtypes of perpetrators: family only, dysphoric–borderline, and generally violent–antisocial men. Another type called 'low level antisocial perpetrators' was added later (Holtzworth-Munroe et al. 2000). These subtypes differed with regard to severity and frequency of the violence, the generality of the violence (only within the family or outside the family), and the perpetrator's psychopathology or emotional dysfunction.

3.3.1.1 Family Only

The family-only (FO) type of perpetrator, or moderately violent offenders are described as least likely to: exert severe and frequent violence; engage in criminal behaviour; use violence outside the home; and display traits of psychopathology or personality disorder. In addition, they are the least likely to have substance abuse issues. The FO perpetrators infrequently engage in DVA consisting of psychological and sexual abuse, and they are the most likely to apologize after being violent. FO perpetrators are inappropriately assertive in their relationship and tend to misinterpret social cues and resort to violence rather than resolving conflicts through other strategies.

3.3.1.2 Dysphoric–Borderline Batterers

The dysphoric–borderline (DB) perpetrators engage in moderate to severe DVA. They are mainly violent toward their intimate partner and may have some degree of involvement in violence outside the home. They may display dysphoric or borderline personality disorder (BPD) related traits. Such perpetrators are also the most psychologically distressed and emotionally volatile and may suffer from delusional jealousy, problems with substance abuse, and a fear of separation from their partners. Their anger is generalized and explosive in nature and is likely to be displayed anytime they become frustrated.

3.3.1.3 Generally Violent and Antisocial Batterers

The third subtype, generally violent and antisocial batterers (GV/A), is described as the most violent category. They engage in a frequent and severe intrafamilial violence, including psychological and sexual abuse. They may also engage repeatedly in severe extrafamilial violence and manifest general criminal behaviour. They are more likely to use weapons and more prone to inflict severe injury on partners and other family members. They are also most likely to be diagnosed with either antisocial personality disorder (APD) or psychopathy, and have alcohol and drug abuse problems.

3.3.1.4 Low Level Antisocial Batterers

Low level antisocial (LLA) batterers fall between the FO and GV/A perpetrator, thus exhibiting moderate extrafamilial as well as intrafamilial violence (Holtzworth-Munroe et al. 2000). They may demonstrate previous registered criminality, although to a lesser extent than the GV/A perpetrator. Furthermore, the LLA perpetrator is unlikely to display psychopathological traits or traits of personality disorder to the same extent as the DB and the GV/A perpetrator (Holtzworth-Munroe et al. 2000).

3.3.2   Jacobson and Gottman's Typology

For their typology, Jacobson and Gottman (1998) examined physiological changes in male perpetrators when they used violence. Jacobson and Gottman (1998) recruited couples via public advertisements and allocated them into groups depending on the pattern of male partner's use of violence. One group ($n = 63$) consisted of perpetrators who exhibited 'low level violence', including perpetrators whose partners reported six or more violent acts—in the past year—such as pushing or slapping, or two or more acts of 'high-level violence', such as kicking or hitting with a fist. The second group ($n = 27$) consisted of men who displayed 'some violence', but insufficient to be classified as 'battering'. The third group ($n = 33$) involved couples dissatisfied with their marriage, but there was no evidence of violence and the fourth group ($n = 20$) involved happily married couples (Jacobson and Gottman 1998). Data was also collected from laboratory observations of non-violent arguments, structured interviews with male perpetrators and their female victims, psychiatric assessment of both partners, and assessment of both partners 'emotional arousal at the physiological level' (heart rate, blood flow, bodily movement, sweating) during an argument. The last stage was videotaped and played back to participants who were asked to describe how they had been feeling at various stages during the argument. Most of these steps were repeated 2 years later to assess relationship stability and use of violence. Jacobson and Gottman (1998) identified two types of perpetrators, including the 'cobras' and 'pit bulls'.

3.3.2.1 Type I Perpetrators: The Cobra

The cobras, who accounted for 20% of perpetrators, exhibited a decrease in heart rate when verbally aggressive and were identified as antisocial, extremely violent, and emotionally abusive (Jacobson and Gottman 1998). They were violent outside their intimate relationship; however, their intimate partners were less likely to leave the relationship. In fact, none of the couples separated 2 years later compared with 50% of the pit bulls whose relationship ended in the same period.

3.3.2.2 Type II Perpetrators: The Pit Bull

Pit bulls were emotionally dependent on their wives and feared 'abandonment'. These men built up their anger during an argument leading to an increased heart rate during an argument. They were likely to have 'jealous rages' and to seek to 'deprive their partners on an independent life' (Jacobson and Gottman 1998: 38). They displayed moderate levels of violence in their intimate relationships, but were less likely to be violent outside their family.

Both types of perpetrators appeared to be controlling as 'the Pit Bulls dominate their wives in any way they can and need control as much as the cobras do, but for different reasons. The Pit Bulls are motivated by a desire to get as much immediate gratification as possible' (Jacobson and Gottman 1998: 38). The cobras appeared to resemble the GV/A male perpetrator, whereas the pit bull resembles the DB perpetrators.

3.4   Typology by Perpetrator: Women

Over the years, there has been a growing recognition that women can also perpetrate violence against their male or female partners (Anderson 2002; Brown 2004; Capaldi et al. 2007; Dasgupta 2002). However, it is also established that women are much more likely to be injured and injured severely than men (Archer 2000; Swan and Snow 2002, 2003).

Researchers attempted to explore, contextualize, and examine the motivations for, and impact of, DVA, especially in response to the higher arrest rate of women in the USA as a result of changes in the mandatory arrest laws (Babcock et al. 2003; Bair-Merritt et al. 2010; Hines and Douglas 2010; Miller and Meloy 2006). Evidence revealed that the ways violence is used by men and women may be different (Miller and Meloy 2006). For instance, men are more likely to use sexual coercion and coercive control against their partners, whereas women's violence is generally less frightening to men (Swan and Snow 2002, 2003). In addition, it is important to understand the role of victimization in understanding the women's motivation to use violence (Swan et al. 2008). In the following, typologies proposed to explain women's use of violence are discussed.

3.4.1 Swan and Snow's Typology

Swan and Snow (2002, 2003) in their research involving 108 DVA perpetrator women, explored women's experience of victimization and perpetration of DVA (physical violence, sexual violence, emotional abuse, injury, and coercive control). Three subtypes were identified: victims, abused aggressors, and mixed relationships (mixed male coercive relation or mixed female coercive relationship).

3.4.1.1 Victims
This type refers to women who were violent, but their partners were not only much more abusive but used more severe violence against them. Thirty-four percent of the sample ($n = 108$) belonged to this category (Swan and Snow 2002). This category was subdivided into two types. The type A male partners committed more of every type of violence than their female counterpart, whereas type B partners committed more severe violence and were coercive against their female partners. However, women committed equal or greater violence and/or emotional abuse against their male counterparts, mainly in self-defence (Swan and Snow 2002, 2003).

3.4.1.2 Aggressor
This category referred to women who were much more abusive than their partners, and accounted for 12% of the study sample. The women exerted both physical abuse and coercive control against their male partner with an intention of retribution and control (Swan and Snow 2003). This category was also divided into two subtypes. The 'type A' women were those who used more of all types of violence against their male partners. The type B women aggressor were those who used greater levels of severe abuse and coercion, but their partner committed equal or more moderate physical and/or emotional abuse.

3.4.1.3 Mixed Relationships
The category consisted of women in mixed relationships and accounted for 50% of the study participants. Thirty-two percent of the women were in a mixed male coercive relationship and 18% of the women were in mixed female coercive relationships (Swan and Snow 2003). The women in mixed male coercive relationships were equally or more violent than their male partners, though the partners were

more coercive than the women themselves. On the other hand, for women in mixed female coercive relationships, women were equally or more coercive than their male partners, but the male partners were more violent than the women.

3.4.2 Miller and Meloy's Typology

Suzanne Miller and Michelle Meloy studied 95 female offenders attending treatment programmes as part of their probation following conviction of DVA (Miller and Meloy 2006). Three categories of abusive women include generalized violent behaviour, frustration response, and defensive behaviour. Women with generalized violent behaviour were generally abusive in and outside family, though they did not exert control over their intimate partners (Miller and Meloy 2006: 98).

Women with frustration response behaviour exhibit abusive behaviour in response to abuse by their partner. This group accounted for 30% of the women in the sample. These women had a history of experiencing abuse from their current or ex intimate partner and these women had responded with violence—unsuccessfully—after trying other measures to stop violence (Miller and Meloy 2006). However, the use of violence by these women did not change their partner's abusive behaviour or the power dynamics in their relationship. Women in the defensive behaviour category used violence as a form of self-defence in situations where they knew their partner was about to become more violent. The group accounted for about 65% of the sample and the majority of them used violence in order to protect their children.

In short, we know about three types of women perpetrator of violence at present. The first group of women uses violence as self-defence. The second group of women uses abuse and exerts power and control in a mutually abusive relationship. The third type consists of women as the primary perpetrators of violence.

Case Study 2
The following case study is a real-life account; however, names and details are changed.

Julie met Garry when he was 22 and she was just 15. The couple married and had two sons together. Their marriage was an abusive one as Garry used to physically and psychologically abuse Julie throughout their marriage. He consistently humiliated her (criticizing her weight and appearance), isolated her from support networks and controlled every aspect of her life. Once, after one of his friends kissed her, Garry anally raped Julie as a punishment. However, he himself repeatedly cheated on Julie. He visited a brothel near where Julie worked. Once away from home, he sent Julie, Christmas card that showed him standing with his Ferrari and two women in bikinis. Julie wasn't allowed to question and even if she tried, Garry would tell her that she was imagining things and that she was 'going mad' and was 'making it all up'.

After 31 years of marriage, they separated, however, they could not live apart so after a year reconciled and planning to live together again. They were planning to raise some funds by selling their house and use the money to take a trip. One morning, Julie went round to meet Garry. Garry asked for breakfast and Julie went out to buy ingredients. Garry, in the meantime, chatted to a woman he had met on a networking website. Julie came back from shopping and before she made him breakfast, she found all information on Garry's phone. She then went on to make and serve breakfast. While Garry was having breakfast, Julie took out the hammer she had in her bag and bludgeoned him with it, hitting him more than 20 times. When she was finished, she stuck a tea towel in his mouth and wrapped his body in old curtains. She wrote a note that read 'I love you, Julie' and placed it on the body, before driving home. It wasn't until the next day, when, called her cousin to confess and then attempted suicide, though suicide prevention team intervened and talked her done.

Time to Reflect
Like previous case study, please examine this case study in relation to various classifications presented. See if all classifications can be applied to this case study? Compare this and previous case study and explore if you can see any differences in terms of perpetration, motivation, or pattern of abuse? How are these two studies similar or different?

3.4.3   So What Does It Mean and Why Does It Matter?

A review of these classifications highlights that not all DVA is the same and that men and women differ in terms of reasons to use their violence and the ways in which they use violence. There are many similarities between various types. For instance, the category of FO perpetrator described by Holtzworth-Munroe and Stuart is similar to Johnson's SCV. The other two types—antisocial and dysphoric—borderline—are similar to CCV (Johnson and Ferraro 2000). CCV and SCV thought to be similar to the Johnston and Campbell's (1993) categories of 'male battering' and 'male-controlling interactive violence', respectively.

In this review, Johnson's typology appears to be the most comprehensive classification which explains the phenomenon of DVA in different circumstances, situations and from varied perspectives. This is supported by another review conducted by Cavanaugh and Gelles (2005) identified three types of perpetrators common in all typology research and these were low, moderate, and high risk offenders. However, much more needs to be explored about the distinction between different typologies and utility of these types (Capaldi and Kim 2007). In addition, we still need to understand: distinctions in the use and motives of violence by men and women, and the potential consequences of different forms of DVA between the genders. We know that women victims of CCV are likely to suffer injuries, manifest symptoms of post-traumatic stress disorder (PTSD), use painkillers, take time off from work, attempt to leave their partner, and seek refuge accommodation on multiple occasion (Johnson and Leone 2005). There is a still a need to explore victims' perspective about different types of DVA (Wangmann 2011) and if the impact of different types of DVA is different on children (Haselschwerdt 2014; Jouriles and McDonald 2015).

Another important methodological concern is about how definition and operationalization coercive control. While coercive control is an overarching issue in abusive relationships, it is often operationalized and measured as a discrete item in addition to other discrete items such as physical, psychological, or sexual abuse. It is also essential to understand the context and the impact of DVA as a lack of such understanding can lead to misidentification of an action. For instance, a woman's threat to leave her partner if he doesn't stop violence can be seen as a control item, rather than an acceptable action (Dutton and Goodman 2005). Understanding the context of an action is important to assess and ascribe meaning to an incident of violence (Dobash and Dobash 2004).

Most typologies put great emphasis on physical violence, but overlook the importance of other forms of DVA. For instance, Johnson's typology only refers to physical abuse and the presence or absence of coercive control. In fact, women who do not experience physical abuse are not identified as DVA victims in Johnson's typology, even when they experience high levels of controlling behaviour (Anderson 2008; Johnson 2008). Similarly, physical violence remains the defining characteristic (Johnston and Campbell 1993; Miller and Meloy 2006).

Another important issue relates to the practical applications of proposed classification and how these can be used in practice by health, social care, and other professionals working in the field of DVA. A study conducted in Australia to explore the use of typologies perceived benefits and challenges associated with the use of DVA typologies by domestic violence practitioners/professionals highlighted a lack of use in practice as the typologies were identified as abstract, risky, and 'unwieldy' to everyday practice (Boxall et al. 2015). Practitioners raised concerns about the unavailability of instruments to help differentiate between classifications, risk of misidentification of violence and compromised the safety of the victim. In addition, it may also be hard to assess abusive experiences that do not fit in with the description of already defined categories. The application and relevance of typologies to different populations is another concern as most research feeding into the development and application of classification comes from western countries and therefore, generalizability and the relevance of these typologies to other countries and context may be limited (Boxall et al. 2015; McPhedran and Baker 2012; Wangmann 2011). As such, the available evidence suggests that the typologies are not much used in clinical and/or professional practice and this mean that typologies are much more theoretical with less practical relevance, something that needs to be explored and developed further.

3.5   Summary

This chapter has provided an overview of the most common perpetrator typologies. The chapter has hopefully helped you understand that DVA perpetrators and their victims represent significantly diverse groups. The chapter highlighted that acknowledging that there may be different typologies of DVA with different reasons, correlates, and consequences and, therefore, differentially appropriate treatment regimens, has the potential to advance not only our definitions and understanding of DVA but also the development and empirical assessment of targeting intervention and preventive approaches.

Summary Points
- Various typologies of classification have been presented to help understand the concept of DVA.
- An understanding of classification of DVA may help develop appropriate empirical assessments, targeted interventions, ways through which such interventions and preventive approaches can be measured effectively.
- Further research is needed to explore if the impact of IPV differs depending on type of IPV.

References

Anderson KL (2002) Perpetrator or victim? Relationships between intimate partner violence and well-being. J Marriage Fam 64(4):851–863

Anderson KL (2008) Is partner violence worse in the context of control? J Marriage Fam 70(5):1157–1168. https://doi.org/10.1111/j.1741-3737.2008.00557.x

Ansara DL, Hindin MJ (2010) Exploring gender differences in the patterns of intimate partner violence in Canada: a latent class approach. J Epidemiol Community Health 64(10):849–854

Ansara DL, Hindin MJ (2011) Psychosocial consequences of intimate partner violence for women and men in Canada. J Interpers Violence 26(8):1628–1645

Archer J (2000) Sex differences in aggression between heterosexual partners: a meta-analytic review. Psychol Bull 126:651–680

Babcock JC, Miller SA, Siard C (2003) Toward a typology of abusive women: differences between partner-only and generally violent women in the use of violence. Psychol Women Q 27(2):153–161. https://doi.org/10.1111/1471-6402.00095

Bair-Merritt MH, Shea Crowne S, Thompson DA, Sibinga E, Trent M, Campbell J (2010) Why do women use intimate partner violence? A systematic review of women's motivations. Trauma Violence Abuse 11(4):178–189. https://doi.org/10.1177/1524838010379003

Beck CJ, Anderson ER, O'Hara KL, Benjamin GAH (2013) Patterns of intimate partner violence in a large, epidemiological sample of divorcing couples. J Fam Psychol 27(5):743

Boxall H, Rosevear L, Payne J (2015) Domestic violence typologies: what value to practice? Trends Issues Crime Criminal Justice (494):1

Brown G (2004) Gender as a factor in the response of the law-enforcement system to violence against partners. Sex Cult 8:3–139

Capaldi DM, Kim HK (2007) Typological approaches to violence in couples: a critique and alternative conceptual approach. Clin Psychol Rev 27(3):253–265

Capaldi D, Kim H, Shortt J (2007) Observed initiation and reciprocity of physical aggression in young, at-risk couples. J Fam Violence 22:101–111

Cavanaugh MM, Gelles RJ (2005) The utility of male domestic violence offender typologies. J Interpers Violence 20:155–166. https://doi.org/10.1177/0886260504268763

Dasgupta SD (2002) A framework for understanding women's use of nonlethal violence in intimate heterosexual relationships. Violence Against Women 8(11):1364–1389. https://doi.org/10.1177/107780102237408

Dobash RP, Dobash RE (2004) Women's violence to men in intimate relationships: working on a puzzle. Br J Criminol 44(3):324–349. https://doi.org/10.1093/bjc/azh026

Dutton M, Goodman L (2005) Coercion in intimate partner violence: toward a new conceptualization. Sex Roles 52(11–12):743–756. https://doi.org/10.1007/s11199-005-4196-6

Eckstein JJ (2017) Intimate terrorism and situational couple violence: classification variability across five methods to distinguish Johnson's violent relationship types. Violence Vict 32(6):955–976

Ellis D, Stuckless N (1996) Mediating and negotiating marital conflicts. Sage, Thousand Oaks

Ellis D, Stuckless N (2006) Separation, domestic violence, and divorce mediation. Conflict Resolution Quarterly 23(4):461–485

Gulliver P, Fanslow JL (2015) The Johnson typologies of intimate partner violence: an investigation of their representation in a general population of New Zealand women. J Child Custody 12(1):25–46

Haselschwerdt ML (2014) Theorizing children's exposure to intimate partner violence using Johnson's typology. J Fam Theory Rev 6(3):199–221

Hines DA, Douglas EM (2010) Intimate terrorism by women towards men: does it exist? J Aggress Confl Peace Res 2(3):36–56. https://doi.org/10.5042/jacpr.2010.0335

Hines D, Brown J, Dunning E (2007) Characteristics of callers to the domestic abuse helpline for men. J Fam Violence 22(2):63–72

Holtzworth-Munroe A, Stuart GL (1994) Typologies of male batterers: three subtypes and the differences among them. Psychol Bull 116:476–497

Holtzworth-Munroe A, Meehan JC, Herron K, Rehman U, Stuart GL (2000) Testing the Holtzworth-Munroe and Stuart (1994) batterer typology. J Consult Clin Psychol 68(6):1000–1019. https://doi.org/10.1037/0022-006X.68.6.1000

Jacobson N, Gottman J (1998) When men batter women: new insights into ending abusive relationships. Simon & Schuster, New York

Johnson MP (1995) Patriarchal terrorism and common couple violence: two forms of violence against women. J Marriage Fam 57(2):283–294. https://doi.org/10.2307/353683

Johnson MP (2000) Conflict and control: images of symmetry and asymmetry in domestic violence. In: Booth ACCA, Clements M (eds) Couples in conflict. Erlbaum, Hillsdale

Johnson MP (2006) Conflict and control: gender symmetry and asymmetry in domestic violence. Violence Against Women 12(11):1003–1018. https://doi.org/10.1177/1077801206293328

Johnson MP (2008) A typology of domestic violence: intimate terrorism, violent resistance and situational couple violence. Northeastern University Press, Lebanon

Johnson MP, Ferraro KJ (2000) Research on domestic violence in the 1990s: making distinctions. J Marriage Fam 62(4):948–963

Johnson MP, Leone JM (2005) The differential effects of intimate terrorism and situational couple violence: findings from the national violence against women survey. J Fam Issues 26(3):322–349. https://doi.org/10.1177/0192513x04270345

Johnston JR, Campbell LEG (1993) A clinical typology of interparental violence in disputed-custody divorces. Am J Orthopsychiatry 63(2):190–199

Jouriles EN, McDonald R (2015) Intimate partner violence, coercive control, and child adjustment problems. J Interpers Violence 30(3):459–474

Kelly JB, Johnson MP (2008) Differentiation among types of intimate partner violence: research update and implications for interventions. Fam Court Rev 46(3):476–499

McKay TE, Lindquist CH, Landwehr J, Ramirez D, Bir A (2018) Postprison relationship dissolution and intimate partner violence: separation-instigated violence or violence-instigated separation? J Offender Rehabil 57(5):294–310

McPhedran S, Baker J (2012) Lethal and non-lethal violence against women in Australia measurement challenges, conceptual frameworks, and limitations in knowledge. Violence Against Women 18(8):958–972

Miller SL, Meloy ML (2006) Women's use of force: voices of women arrested for domestic violence. Violence Against Women 12(1):89–115. https://doi.org/10.1177/1077801205277356

Swan SC, Snow DL (2002) A typology of women's use of violence in intimate relationships. Violence Against Women 8(3):286–319. https://doi.org/10.1177/107780120200800302

Swan SC, Snow DL (2003) Behavioral and psychological differences among abused women who use violence in intimate relationships. Violence Against Women 9(1):75–109. https://doi.org/10.1177/1077801202238431

Swan SC, Gambone LJ, Caldwell JE, Sullivan TP, Snow DL (2008) A review of research on women's use of violence with male intimate partners. Violence Vict 23(3):301

Tanha M, Beck CJA, Figueredo AJ, Raghavan C (2010) Sex differences in intimate partner violence and the use of coercive control as a motivational factor for intimate partner violence. J Interpers Violence 25(10):1836–1854. https://doi.org/10.1177/0886260509354501

Walker LE (1984) The battered woman syndrome. Springer, New York

Wangmann JM (2011) Different types of intimate partner violence—an exploration of the literature. http://www.adfvc.unsw.edu.au/PDF%20files/IssuesPaper_22.pdf

Yllö K, Bograd M (1988) Feminist perspectives on wife abuse. Sage, Newbury Park

Clinical Settings Where Domestic Violence and Abuse May Be Encountered

4

Michaela Rogers

4.1 Introduction

There is a growing body of work exploring domestic violence and abuse (DVA) in relation to primary and secondary healthcare settings and fields of practice. This is unsurprising as it has become increasingly apparent that it is practitioners in health services (General Practitioners (GPs), health visitors, emergency and ambulance staff, midwives, and sexual health practitioners) who are often the very first point of contact for people suffering from abuse. Not only this, it is frequently reported by survivors of DVA that healthcare practitioners are those professionals that they would be most likely to speak to about their experiences (Department of Health 2005; Ahmad et al. 2017). However, the health sector has been described as a relatively 'late entrant' into the response to DVA (Laing and Humphreys 2013: 126). Despite this, effective recognition, management, and pathways to support are now acknowledged to be key priorities for healthcare settings (McGarry and Ali 2016).

This chapter starts with an overview of the professional standards and policies that apply in clinical settings. It is noted, however, that whilst there is a growing recognition of the importance of the effective management of DVA within these settings at a policy level, overall, frontline healthcare professionals are not adequately prepared and equipped to effectively respond to victims-survivors of DVA who present in healthcare settings (Taylor et al. 2013). The importance of training and education is subsequently explored to contextualise the work required in healthcare settings in relation to screening for and responding to DVA. Whilst acknowledging that there are various areas of healthcare practice (including minor injury units, and sexual health clinics) that are relevant to this discussion, four are highlighted in this chapter as typical settings where practitioners will encounter

M. Rogers (✉)
Department of Sociological Studies, University of Sheffield, Sheffield, UK
e-mail: m.rogers@sheffield.ac.uk

© Springer Nature Switzerland AG 2020
P. Ali, J. McGarry (eds.), *Domestic Violence in Health Contexts: A Guide for Healthcare Professions*, https://doi.org/10.1007/978-3-030-29361-1_4

victims-survivors of DVA. These are general practice, midwifery and antenatal care, emergency departments and mental health. The discussion will illuminate the divergences in responding to DVA across these four fields of healthcare.

4.2   Professional Standards and Codes of Practice

The need for professional standards and codes of practice in relation to the management of DVA is clear. This is especially important as healthcare professionals are tasked with responsibilities and duties in working with children and adults considered to be vulnerable including where abuse and maltreatment is present. Moreover, in the UK for example, there are legislative frameworks that reinforce this duty. For children, it is reflected in the policy guidance *Working Together to Safeguard Children* (Department of Education 2018) and in the case of vulnerable adults, the responsibilities and duties around welfare and safeguarding are set out in the document *Safeguarding Vulnerable People in the NHS: Accountability and Assurance Framework* (NHS England 2015). These documents are not specifically targeted at addressing DVA but cover abuse and neglect in its various forms (including child maltreatment and elder abuse).

These policies do indicate, however, that addressing DVA is a key national priority and driver in the UK. Underpinning all policy and practice responses should be the principles and ethos set out in the *Ending Violence against Women and Girls Strategy 2016–2020* (EVAWG) (Home Office 2016). This strategy states that tackling DVA is 'everyone's responsibility' and a commitment in this regard should be reflected across the public sector (Home Office 2016: 11). The EVAWG strategy has three key target areas which are prevention, early help, and increased reporting. These strategic objectives, along with a commitment to enhance interagency collaboration, can be found at a policy level for all health and social care professionals. This is reflected in the National Institute for Health and Care Excellence (NICE) guidance, *Domestic violence and abuse: How health services, social care and the organisations they work with can respond effectively*, published in 2014. The NICE guidance has influenced the development of policy and guidance to address DVA across healthcare settings. For example, the objectives set out in the NICE guidance underpin the revised document *Responding to domestic abuse: A resource for health professionals* (Department of Health 2017). This document aims to support continuing improvement in the response from health and care services as well as from allied healthcare partners.

The Department of Health resource details those indicators that should help practitioners to recognise the signs and symptoms of DVA and to, therefore, identify potential victims. It guides practitioners to initiate routine enquiry and respond sensitively and effectively to disclosures of abuse. In tandem, this document and the EVAWG strategy are working to strengthen the role of healthcare services and practitioners. In addition, various disciplines in healthcare have distinct codes of practice and standards which are targeted at the profession and specifically address DVA. For example, the Royal College of Nursing (RCN) has a dedicated *Risk*

Assessment Pathway to identify Domestic Abuse and a *Position Statement on Domestic Abuse* (RCN 2019). The Nursing and Midwifery Council's (NMC 2015) code for nurses and midwives states that nurses should respect and uphold human rights, putting the interests of people using services first, making care and safety a priority, and recognising, assessing, and responding to physical, social, and psychological needs. This clearly implicates nurses and midwives in the professional response to tackling DVA.

Professional bodies with a global, as opposed to national, remit have also recognised the problem of DVA as entrenched and endemic (WHO 2017). For instance, in 1996 (amended in 2010) the World Medical Association (WMA) issued a statement on family violence together with a resolution on violence against women and girls (WMA 2010). In this statement, family violence incorporates DVA, honour killings, and child marriage to name a few. In addition to making recommendations directed at clinicians dealing with abuse cases, through this statement, the WMA urges national medical associations to press for change via an interagency approach identifying two actions: to facilitate the coordination of action and interventions addressing DVA; and to enable research to enhance understandings about the prevalence, risk factors, outcomes, and appropriate care for victims-survivors.

Time to Reflect
Can you think of the reasons why different areas of healthcare practice might need individualised professional standards and protocols for responding to DVA? What are the benefits and limitations of these?

4.3 Education, Training, and Awareness

Whilst professional standards provide the formal framework for healthcare professionals, these are of limited use without an awareness of DVA and the expertise in knowing how to respond to it. Education and training on DVA for healthcare professionals builds knowledge, improves attitudes and results in increased confidence to recognise and respond to abuse appropriately (Litherland 2012; Sundborg et al. 2012). It has been suggested that interprofessional education is best practice in this regard as, in addition to generating greater knowledge and awareness, it enhances understandings about the value and function of an interagency approach and generates shared understandings of DVA and the needs of victims-survivors (Leppäkoski et al. 2015). This is congruent with the recommendations of global and national policies and drivers as noted earlier (WMA 2010; NICE 2014; Home Office 2016).

The impact of education and training in the context of DVA awareness can be limited by organisational cultures and support however (Husso et al. 2012). This support (or lack thereof) can be embedded in organisational infrastructure (through appropriate policy and protocols) but shown in other ways too, for example, by having a DVA nurse specialist and successful and routine interagency collaboration (Litherland 2012; Sundborg et al. 2012; McGarrry and Nairn 2015). The danger of having individuals who champion issues such as DVA, however, is that the responsibility often falls to those people who already have an interest in the issue without the full support of teams or wider organisational structures. Additionally, the WHO (2010) emphasises that *all* healthcare professionals should be equipped, through regulation and appropriate training, to recognise and respond to DVA.

4.4 Screening and Routine Inquiry in Healthcare Settings

A systematic review of existing research was carried out to ascertain whether routine screening in healthcare settings was beneficial and it found that whilst screening increases identification of victims-survivors, there is insufficient evidence to justify screening in healthcare settings (O'Doherty et al. 2015). This does not indicate that screening should not take place, rather this review highlights the gap in current knowledge about how best to screen and in which healthcare settings. A study by Husso et al. (2012) highlighted barriers to routine screening and responses in healthcare settings. They identified four key 'frames', or viewpoints, that nurses adopted when conceptualising DVA as it presented in their work setting. These viewpoints were:

- A practical frame: where there was no time to deal with non-medical issues and nurses did not know where to refer
- A medical frame: where DVA was considered to be a social issue and not a nurse's responsibility
- A psychological frame: where the issue was avoided
- An individualistic frame: where DVA was viewed as an individual's problem

These frames, or viewpoints, were compounded by confusion as to whose role it is to intervene (Husso et al. 2012; Williston and Lafreniere 2013) and by the complexity of victims-survivors who commonly conceal their experiences (Litherland 2012; Bradbury-Jones et al. 2014). This suggests that screening cannot happen without awareness and training, but training alone is inadequate as a means of enabling better recognition or enhancing practice (Ritchie et al. 2013; LoGiudice 2015). This is highlighted by Sundborg et al. (2012) who argued that even when nurses identify DVA, there can be a tendency to prioritise medical issues and treatment and to avoid screening for DVA. This can result from organisational cultures which means that responding to DVA is avoided in favour of other priorities or demands. There are many additional reasons including: lack of time and/or resources; limited knowledge; uncertainty about role and responsibility; fear of risks to both the practitioner and patient (Husso et al. 2012; Litherland 2012; Williston and Lafreniere 2013; Bradbury-Jones et al. 2014; Ahmad et al. 2017).

Bradbury-Jones et al. (2014) explored DVA awareness and recognition in primary healthcare professionals (*n* = 29) and female victims-survivors (*n* = 14). The women in the study articulated a desire to be asked about DVA. The study suggested that it is the remit and responsibility of healthcare professionals to create a supportive environment to facilitate such inquiries. This does require skill as the environment should promote a therapeutic relationship to develop, enabling an open discussion enhanced by use of 'guided conversation support tools' (Bradbury-Jones et al. 2014: 3065). Unsurprisingly, Bradbury-Jones et al. (2014) found that the more experienced or prepared healthcare professionals are for identifying and screening for DVA, the more likely they are to recognise and screen for it in future. Allen (2013: 92) argues that existing studies clearly indicate what women want from healthcare professionals which is:

- Before disclosure or routine questioning, to consider how to ensure continuity of care.
- To create an environment that is safe so that it is possible for women to disclose current and/or past abuse.
- When the issue of abuse is disclosed, be careful not to pressure women to fully disclose.
- To be careful to ensure that women feel that they have control over the situation but to simultaneously address any immediate safety issues.
- That in later consultations, try to understand the chronic nature of the problem and ensure that support is followed up.

The WHO (2010) states that healthcare professionals should be confident in asking direct questions when women present in specific circumstances including with: anxiety, depression, or substance misuse; sexually transmitted infections or other recurrent gynaecological symptoms; and during the course of antenatal care.

4.5   General Practice (GP) Settings

The statistic that one in four women will experience DVA at some point in their lifetime is long-established (Refuge 2017) but in GP settings, the lifetime prevalence for women is claimed to be greater reaching as high as one in three (Feder et al. 2009). Historically, healthcare professionals at GP settings have not routinely asked questions about DVA and it is a topic that many feel nervous or too fearful to broach (Yeung et al. 2012). Yet the consultation that occurs when an individual visits their GP is the 'cornerstone' of general practice and offers the perfect opportunity to do so (Denness 2013). As noted earlier, the WHO (2010) states that healthcare professionals should be confident in asking questions about DVA and GPs should ask when patients present with pain (specific or unspecified), headaches, tiredness, low mood/depression, anxiety, gastrointestinal complaints, and gynaecological; all of which are common symptoms, or cues, in victims-survivors (Feder and Howarth 2014; Valpied and Hegarty 2015).

The value of responding to DVA in primary healthcare, and particularly by GPs, is now recognised and there has been a proliferation of studies into the role that primary healthcare professionals can play (García-Moreno et al. 2014; Dowrick et al. 2018). In the UK, there has been a very specific shift in the response to DVA within general practice as a result of the development and commissioning of the

Identification and Referral to Improve Safety (IRIS) programme. IRIS is specifically designed for general practice settings and it offers a programme of training
and support to facilitate greater recognition and referral. Core areas of IRIS are
training and education, clinical enquiry, care pathways, and an enhanced referral
pathway to specialist DVA support. The programme was tested in a randomised
controlled trial (Feder et al. 2011). IRIS has resulted in greater collaboration
between primary care and third sector organisations specialising in DVA as an advocate educator (employed by the DVA service) is linked to a general practice.
Subsequently, there is a more streamlined pathway from referral to intervention.
The success of IRIS is reflected in the EVAWG strategy and action plan which states
that there should be a government action to 'support improvements in responses of
health professionals to VAWG for example through roll out of the IRIS programme'
(Home Office 2016: 53). Box 4.1 highlights an example of how IRIS has helped to
improve identification of and responses to DVA in one GP surgery.

4.6   Pregnancy and Midwifery

Pregnancy can be either a trigger or an escalator for DVA and nearly one in three
women who suffer from DVA during their lifetime report that the first incidence of
violence happened whilst they were pregnant (Lewis and Drife 2001). Worldwide,
the prevalence of DVA during pregnancy ranges from approximately 2–13.5%
(Devries et al. 2010). Whilst the perpetration of abuse during pregnancy can resemble the types of maltreatment experienced by victims-survivors who are not pregnant, there can be very distinct and targeted acts of violence that are directed at a
woman's pregnancy such as blows and kicks to the abdomen or very brutal acts of
being stamped or jumped upon on the abdomen (Edin et al. 2010). Pregnant women
can be coerced and forced to engage in negative behaviours that are harmful to a
foetus (such as smoking, alcohol, and/or substance use) or prevented from attending
antenatal checks and care.

Box 4.1 Case Study: Rita
Fifty-eight-year-old Rita has been married to Thomas for 27 years. They have
two adult children, Michael and Catherine. When Rita was 33 she lost a baby
through stillbirth. Rita had been seeing her GP, Dr. McNeish, for a number of
years due to long-standing mental health conditions, anxiety and depression.
Recently, she has been feeling very tired and put it down to her recently diagnosed COPD. She also has frequent headaches. All conditions are generally
manageable with existing medication.
    In 2016, the local Clinical Commissioning Group decided to commission
IRIS as a trial in response to concerns about the scale of DVA in the locality.
Dr. McNeish's practice became part of the trial. Members of the practice

undertook training which was delivered by an advocate educator employed by the local DVA organisation.

An important feature of commissioning IRIS results in having software installed into the general practice. This provides an electronic prompt in medical records; this pop-up is called HARKS. HARKS stands for: Humiliate, Afraid, Rape, Kick, and Safety and is linked to health symptoms of DVA (Howell and Johnson 2011). HARKS is:

- A practical reminder to clinicians to ask about DVA
- A flagging system noting HARK+ on the patient record when there is a positive disclosure of DVA
- A safety tool instructing clinicians to assess immediate risk

When Dr. McNeish next saw Rita she was still complaining of tiredness and her headaches were becoming more frequent. The HARKS pop-up prompted Dr. McNeish to ask Rita about her relationship with Thomas. Rita opened up to him and admitted that she'd been experiencing DVA from Thomas since the start of their marriage. The abuse was physical, sexual, and psychological at first. In the last 15 years, it had been mostly psychological and emotional abuse, but relentless. Rita was able to access support for the first time via the advocate educator. She attended support sessions at the general practice so Thomas was not suspicious.

As previously highlighted in Chap. 1, DVA during pregnancy is associated with adverse health impacts for both mother and foetus (Finnbogadóttir and Dykes 2016). A systematic literature review of interventions for women in pregnancy who are victims of DVA found that counselling was considered to be useful as was mentoring albeit there is a modest evidence-base in this regard (Leneghan et al. 2012). A study by Salmon et al. (2013) sought to explore the acceptability of antenatal enquiry, as an intervention, from the perspective of women using maternity services. It also sought to understand the experiences of referral and support offered to women who had positively disclosed abuse. Salmon et al. found that out of the 236 survey responses, 94.4% indicated that they felt comfortable with a midwife asking about abuse. In addition, 96.6% indicated that it was appropriate for a midwife to ask and that midwives should be able to respond to positive disclosure.

There are, however, more barriers for women with additional needs in respect of accessing support through antenatal care *and* DVA support. In addition, there can be delays in accessing antenatal care in abusive contexts. For instance, a systematic review of the available literature for women with disabilities found that for women with a mental health diagnosis, poor relationships with healthcare professionals, in addition to other challenges, was a barrier to a woman's utilisation of maternity services (Breckenridge et al. 2014). The study also found that delayed and inadequate care has adverse effects on women's physical and psychological health yet only one study in their review identified strategies currently being used to improve access to services for disabled women experiencing abuse (Breckenridge et al. 2014). Access is a two-way process, however, and the barriers encountered by practitioners have also been explored in research. For example, a study by LoGiudice (2015: 7) found that healthcare providers are cognisant of the benefits of prenatal screening for DVA but 'do not routinely screen given the barriers of partners being present, variations in timing and manner of addressing DVA, and feel "lost in the maze" of disclosure'.

Time to Reflect
Consider the concept of feeling 'lost in the maze' of disclosure. What does this mean to you? How do you think healthcare providers can overcome such challenges to practice that routinely involves asking about abuse?

4.7   Emergency Departments

There is increasing evidence showing that a considerable number of people attend emergency departments (EDs) as a result of DVA (Boyle et al. 2006; Ahmad et al. 2017). When making any claims using statistics that portray the scale of DVA, it is important to note that there are limitations in accurately measuring prevalence rates. This applies to presentations in EDs for various reasons, such as lack of full disclosures or inaccurate/absent recording (Boyle et al. 2010). Moreover, research suggests that detection rates of DVA are low in emergency departments (Timmis et al. 2010) with earlier research indicating a cultural barrier as professionals based in EDs had questioned the appropriateness of ED resources in screening for DVA (Dowd et al. 2002). However, there is an emerging evidence-base which is building a picture of DVA and EDs. For instance, findings in an international study found that 44% of domestic homicide victims had visited an ED in the 2 years preceding their death (Wadman and Muelleman 1999). In addition, it is recognised that there are important differences in women experiencing DVA who present at EDs compared to other women (Ansari and Boyle 2017) including higher prevalence rates of alcohol and substance misuse as well as psychiatric/psychological issues such as self-harm (Boyle et al. 2006; Sutherland et al. 2013).

Ansari and Boyle (2017) highlight that for those victims-survivors presenting to an ED with repetitive and non-specific ailments, this may be the only point of contact between them and professionals. In addition, the relative anonymity of ED may mean that victims-survivors choose to access an ED rather than any other health or care provision. As such, this attendance may represent a critical window in which practitioners are able to screen for and respond to DVA. Importantly, there is a growing evidence-base exploring the potential for professionals based in EDs to respond to DVA in this regard. One study set out to determine whether training and the provision of specialist documentation led to improved assessment of female victims of DVA presenting to an ED (Ritchie et al. 2013). The researchers found that training alone did not lead to change. Rather, what did help was introducing specialist documentation in addition to training as this was associated with an improvement in the assessment of female victims-survivors (Ritchie et al. 2013). However, it has also been identified that this type of screening process for ED professionals has limited benefit without a wider, supportive organisational infrastructure (McGarry and Nairn 2015).

In terms of the narratives of victims-survivors of DVA who attend EDs, Yam (2000: 469) found that female victims-survivors reported to experience a 'rushed and hurried approach' from staff which reinforced any fear or hesitancy in making disclosures. Yam's finding is reflected in other literature as ED staff have reported that time is a barrier to effectively responding to DVA and the cultures of EDs have been depicted as fast-paced with quick interventions which similarly prevents disclosures of DVA (Andersson et al. 2012; McGarry and Nairn 2015). Whilst there is a lack of standardisation in terms of how EDs should respond to and manage DVA, it is clear that the restrictions imposed by time and the pace of work is an issue in EDs as any response to a sensitive issue such as DVA does require time and pace that is dictated by the victim-survivor and not the practice setting. However, in the UK, there have been positive reports where independent domestic violence advocates (a role offering specialist support for higher risk DVA victims-survivors) have been based in EDs and findings from an evaluation of a DVA specialist nurse located in an ED were favourable albeit with some persisting limitations around the issues already noted here and in relation to feelings of 'helplessness' across ED teams more generally (McGarrry and Nairn 2015: 69). On an individual level, this helplessness was tied to levels of confidence and knowledge highlighting the ongoing needs for training, dedicated resources, and culture change to enable ED staff to respond efficiently and appropriately to DVA. In Chap. 4, we return to the ED setting within the context of the discussion surrounding screening and enquiry within healthcare contexts.

4.8 Mental Health

There is clear evidence of the negative consequences of DVA on mental health for victims-survivors across the life course (Stöckl and Penhale 2015). Studies have shown that the experience of DVA affects low self-esteem as well as increasing depressive symptoms, post-traumatic stress disorder (PTSD), and suicidal ideation (von Eye and Bogat 2006; Howard et al. 2010). Exposure to DVA as a child can result in mental health problems in childhood, adolescence, and adulthood (Herrenkohl et al. 2008). As such, the evidence shows that there are more short- and long-term mental health effects for victims-survivors than for non-abused women (Stöckl and Penhale 2015 as described in Chap. 1. Additionally, there are some psychological indicators that healthcare professionals can be alert to. These are: insomnia; depression; suicidal ideation; PTSD; eating disorders; substance misuse; and symptoms of anxiety, panic disorder or somatoform disorder (where physical symptoms present that cannot be attributed to an organic disease and appear to be of psychological origin) (Hegarty and O'Doherty 2011). A study conducted in Spain found that PTSD is the most frequently found mental health condition in victims-survivors with a mean prevalence of 64% in abused women (Pico-Alfonso 2005). The symptoms of PTSD can have a significant impact on daily life and the ability to perform daily living activities. These symptoms can develop soon after a traumatic event but, in a minority of cases, there may be a delay of months or even years before symptoms appear. The appearance and everyday impact of symptoms can vary from being manageable to debilitating. Symptoms generally take the form of these categories:

- Re-experiencing: This is the most typical symptom of PTSD and involves a person having experiences linked to the traumatic events such as vivid flashbacks, nightmares, repetitive or distressing images/sensations or physical sensations such as pain, sweating, nausea, or trembling.
- Avoidance/emotional numbing: This is when people try to avoid thinking about the traumatic event and this involves blocking out the memory. Some will try to address their feelings by trying to not feel anything at all (termed 'emotional numbing') which can lead to people becoming withdrawn and isolated.
- Hyperarousal: High levels of arousal or anxiety can be experienced as a symptom meaning that a person finds it difficult to relax. This means that a person can be irritable, prone to angry outbursts and experience challenges to their concentration and sleeping.

PTSD is a complex condition and can be present in many other ways. It can include other mental health problems (phobias, obsessive compulsive disorders, and depression) as well as self-harming or destructive behaviours (use of substances). Physical symptoms (such as headaches, dizziness, and chest pains) are common too. There are associated negative outcomes related to PTSD such as poor decision-making, inconsistent parenting, and behaviour dysfunction among offspring (Symes et al. 2018). Studies which have explored the presence of PTSD in victims-survivors have found that whilst all forms of abuse can be identified, it is the degree of psychological abuse (coercive control, intimation, manipulation, and so on) which appear to be a strong indicator for higher levels of PTSD and depression (Cascardi et al. 1999).

Whilst there is a considerable evidence-base exploring the interconnection of mental health and DVA, there is not the equivalent body of work which explores responses to DVA in mental health settings. It has been reported that traditionally in mental health settings, practitioners have tended to avoid suspicions of abuse to focus on the mental health issue (Humphreys and Thiara 2003). A review of literature focusing on the recognition of DVA in mental health nursing found only two research papers that met their inclusion criteria (Byrom et al. 2017). One of these studies (see Nyame et al. 2013) constituted a cross-sectional survey of 81 psychiatrists and 50 community mental health nurses in London. Rates of universal screening were found to be low at 15%. Nyame et al. found that psychiatrists were more likely than mental health nurses to provide information to service users, but mental health nurses were more likely to undertake assessment and management of DVA. However, a high proportion of respondents had inadequate knowledge of services available. Given that people with mental health conditions are more likely to be survivors of DVA, and vice versa (Howard et al. 2013), it can be argued that mental health services have a major role to play in tackling DVA (Oram et al. 2017). This has important implications for mental health practitioners and clinicians.

4.9   Summary

This chapter provided an overview of the policy framework that guides healthcare professionals in a variety of clinical settings when encountering people affected by DVA. In doing so it has illuminated the joint responsibilities and roles that healthcare professionals have and shared protocols and ethics in operation (whilst acknowledging that there will be additional, more localised policies and procedures). An underpinning framework to professional standards and ethics has value in an environment where tackling DVA is 'everyone's responsibility' (Home Office 2016). The importance of training and knowledge were explored in relation to screening practices and routine inquiry in healthcare settings. Finally, the chapter ends by putting the spotlight on four areas of practice: general practice; antenatal care; emergency department care; and mental health. This illustrates the imbalance in current responses to DVA across the healthcare sector. It draws attention to the need for further research and evidence-based interventions for all healthcare settings.

Summary Points
- Healthcare professionals may encounter DVA in many different healthcare settings.
- It is important for healthcare professionals to understand the policy frameworks underpinning the response to victims-survivors of DVA.
- There are many different factors that may have an impact on healthcare professional's ability to support DVA victim-survivor in clinical settings.

Web Resources

NICE (2014) Domestic violence and abuse: multi-agency working. https://www.nice.org.uk/Guidance/PH50
Department of Health (2017) Responding to domestic abuse A resource for health professionals. https://www.gov.uk/government/publications/domestic-abuse-a-resource-for-health-professionals
Department of Education (2018) Working together to safeguard children: a guide to inter-agency working to safeguard and promote the welfare of children. https://assets.publishing.service.gov.uk/government/uploads/system/uploads/attachment_data/file/779401/Working_Together_to_Safeguard-Children.pdf

References

Ahmad I, Ali PA, Rehman S, Talpur A, Dhingra K (2017) Intimate partner violence screening in emergency department: a rapid review of the literature. J Clin Nurs 26(21-22):3271–3285

Allen M (2013) Social work and intimate partner violence. Routledge, Abingdon

Andersson H, Jakobsson E, Furaker C, Nilsson K (2012) The everyday work at a Swedish emergency department; the practitioner's perspective. Int Emerg Nurs 20:58–68

Ansari S, Boyle A (2017) Emergency department-based interventions for women suffering domestic abuse: a critical literature review. Eur J Emerg Med 14(1):13–18

Boyle A, Jones P, Lloyd S (2006) The association between domestic violence and self harm in emergency medicine patients. Emerg Med J 23:604–607

Boyle A, Frith C, Edgcumbe D, McDougall C (2010) What factors are associated with repeated domestic assault in patients attending an emergency department? A cohort study. Emerg Med J 27:203–206

Bradbury-Jones C, Taylor J, Kroll T, Duncan F (2014) Domestic abuse awareness and recognition among primary healthcare professionals and abused women: a qualitative investigation. J Clin Nurs 23(21–22):3057–3068

Breckenridge JP, Devaney J, Kroll T, Lazenbatt A, Taylor J, Bradbury-Jones C (2014) Access and utilisation of maternity care for disabled women who experience domestic abuse: a systematic review. BMC Pregnancy Childbirth 14:234

Byrom B, Collier E, Rogers M (2017) Nurses' recognition of domestic violence and abuse. Br J Mental Health Nurs 6(6). https://doi-org.sheffield.idm.oclc.org/10.12968/bjmh.2017.6.6.286

Cascardi M, O'Leary KD, Schee KA (1999) Co-occurrence and correlates of posttraumatic stress disorder and major depression in physically abused women. J Fam Violence 14:227–247

Denness C (2013) What are consultation models for? InnovAiT: Education and Inspiration for General Practice 6(9):592–599

Department of Education (2018) Working together to safeguard children: a guide to inter-agency working to safeguard and promote the welfare of children. DoE, London

Department of Health (2005) Responding to domestic abuse: a handbook for health professionals. DoH, London

Department of Health (2017) Responding to domestic abuse a resource for health professionals. DoH, London

Devries KM, Kishor S, Johnson H, Stöckl H, Bacchus LJ, García-Moreno C, Watts C (2010) Intimate partner violence during pregnancy: analysis of prevalence data from 19 countries. Reprod Health Matters 18(36):158–170

Dowd M, Kennedy C, Knapp J, Stallbaumer-Rouyer J (2002) Mothers' and health care providers' perspectives on screening for intimate partner violence in a pediatric emergency department. Arch Pediatr Adolesc Med 156:794–799

Dowrick A, Sohal A, Kelly M, Griffiths C, Feder G (2018) Domestic violence: safe and compassionate consultations. InnovAiT: Education and Inspiration for General Practice 11(4):218–225

Edin K, Dahlren L, Lalos A, Hogberg U (2010) 'Keeping up a front': narratives about intimate partner violence, pregnancy, and antenatal care. Violence Against Women 16:180–206

Feder G, Howarth E (2014) The epidemiology of gender based violence. In: Bewley S, Welch J (eds) ABC of domestic and sexual violence. Oxford, Wiley-Blackwell, pp 30–36

Feder G, Ramsay J, Dunne D, Rose M, Arsene C, Norman R, Taket A (2009) How far does screening women for domestic (partner) violence in different health-care settings meet the UK National Screening Committee criteria for a screening programme? Systematic reviews of nine UK National Screening Committee criteria. Health Technol Assess 13(16):iii–iv, xi–xiii, 1–113, 137–347. https://doi.org/10.3310/hta13160

Feder G, Agnew Davies R, Baird K, Dunne D, Eldridge S, Griffiths C, Gregory A, Howell A, Johnson M, Ramsay J, Rutterford C, Sharp D (2011) Identification and referral to improve safety (IRIS) of women experiencing domestic violence with a primary care training and support programme: a cluster randomised controlled trial. Lancet 378(9805):1788–1795. https://doi.org/10.1016/S0140-6736(11)61179-3

Finnbogadóttir H, Dykes A (2016) Increasing prevalence and incidence of domestic violence during the pregnancy and one and half year postpartum, as well as risk factors: a longitudinal cohort study in southern Sweden. BMC Pregnancy Childbirth 16(1):327

García-Moreno C, Hegarty K, Lucas d'Oliveira AF, Koziol-MacLain J, Colombini M, Feder G (2014) The health-systems response to violence against women. Lancet 385(9977):1567–1579

Hegarty K, O'Doherty L (2011) Intimate partner violence: identification and response in general practice. Aust Fam Physician 40(11):852–856

Herrenkohl TI, Sousa C, Tajima EA, Herrenkohl RC, Moylan CA (2008) Intersection of child abuse and children's exposure to domestic violence. Trauma Violence Abuse 9:84–99

Home Office (2016) Ending violence against women and girls: strategy 2016–2020. https://www.gov.uk/government/uploads/system/uploads/attachment_data/file/522166/VAWG_Strategy_FINAL_PUBLICATION_MASTER_vRB.PDF

Howard LM, Trevillion K, Agnew-Davies R (2010) Domestic violence and mental health. Int Rev Psychiatry 22:525–534

Howard LM, Agnew-Davies R, Feder G (2013) Domestic violence and mental health. RCPsych Publications, London

Howell A, Johnson M (2011) Commissioning guidance: the IRIS solution—responding to domestic violence and abuse in general practice. The University of Bristol, Bristol

Humphreys C, Thiara R (2003) Mental health and domestic violence: I call it symptoms of abuse. Br J Soc Work 33:209–226

Husso N, Virkki T, Norko M, Holma J, Laitila A, Mäntysaari M (2012) Making sense of domestic violence intervention in professional health care. Health Soc Care Community 20(2):347–355

Laing L, Humphreys C (2013) Social work and domestic violence: developing critical and reflective practice. Sage, London

Leneghan S, Gillen P, Sinclair M (2012) Interventions to reduce domestic abuse in pregnancy: a qualitative systematic review. Evid Based Midwifery 10(4):137–142

Leppäkoski TH, Flinck A, Paavilainen E (2015) Grater commitment to the domestic violence training is required. J Interprof Care 29(3):281–283

Lewis G, Drife J (2001) Why mothers die: report from the confidential enquiries into maternal deaths in the UK 1997–9. RCOG Press, London

Litherland R (2012) The health visitor's role in the identification of domestic abuse. Community Pract 85(8):20–23

LoGiudice JA (2015) Pre-natal screening for intimate partner violence: a qualitative meta-synthesis. Appl Nurs Res 28(1):2–9

McGarrry J, Nairn S (2015) An exploration of the perceptions of emergency department nursing staff towards the role of a domestic abuse nurse specialist: a qualitative study. Int Emerg Nurs 23(2):65–70

McGarry J, Ali P (2016) Researching domestic violence and abuse in healthcare settings: challenges and issues. J Res Nurs 21(5):465–476

NHS England (2015) Safeguarding vulnerable people in the NHS—accountability and assurance framework. https://www.england.nhs.uk/wp-content/uploads/2015/07/safeguarding-accountability-assurance-framework.pdf. Accessed 12 Apr 2019

NICE (2014) Domestic violence and abuse: how health services, social care and the organisations they work with can respond effectively. NICE, London

Nursing and Midwifery Council (2015) The code: professional standards of practice and behaviour for nurses and midwives. NMC, London

Nyame S, Howard LM, Feder G, Trevillion K (2013) A survey of mental health professionals' knowledge, attitudes and preparedness to respond to domestic violence. J Ment Health 22(6):536–543

O'Doherty L, Hegarty K, Ramsay J, Davidson LL, Feder G, Taft A (2015) Screening women for intimate partner violence in healthcare settings. Cochrane Database Syst Rev (7):CD007007. https://doi.org/10.1002/14651858.CD007007.pub3

Oram S, Khalifeh H, Howard LM (2017) Violence against women and mental health. Lancet Psychiatry 4(2):159–170

Pico-Alfonso MA (2005) Psychological intimate partner violence: the major predictor of posttrau-matic stress disorder in abused women. Neurosci Biobehav Rev 29:181–193

RCN (2019) Domestic abuse: professional resources. https://www.rcn.org.uk/clinical-topics/domestic-violence-and-abuse/professional-resources. Accessed 12 Apr 2019

Refuge (2017) The facts. https://www.refuge.org.uk/our-work/forms-of-violence-and-abuse/domestic-violence/domestic-violence-the-facts/

Ritchie M, Nelson K, Wills R, Jones L (2013) Does training and documentation improve emergency department assessments of domestic violence victims? J Fam Violence 28:471–477

Salmon D, Baird KM, White P (2013) Women's views and experiences of antenatal enquiry for domestic abuse during pregnancy. Health Expect 18(5):867–878

Stöckl H, Penhale B (2015) Intimate partner violence and its association with physical and mental health symptoms among older women in Germany. J Interpers Violence 30(17):3089–3111

Sundborg EM, Saleh-Stattin N, Wändell P, Törnkvist L (2012) Nurses' preparedness to care for women exposed to intimate partner violence: a quantitative study in primary health care. BMC Nurs 11(1):1–11

Sutherland MA, Fantasia HC, McClain N (2013) Abuse experiences, substance use, and reproductive health in women seeking care at an emergency department. J Emerg Nurs 39(4):325–333

Symes L, McFarlane J, Maddoux J, Levine LB, Landrum KS, McFarlane CD (2018) Establishing concurrent validity for a brief PTSD screen among women in a domestic violence shelter. J Interpers Violence. https://doi.org/10.1177/0886260518779595

Taylor J, Bradbury-Jones C, Kroll T, Duncan F (2013) Health professionals' beliefs about domestic abuse and the issue of disclosure: a critical incident technique study. Health Soc Care Community 21(5):489–499

Timmis S, Olimpio C, Hann G, Daniels J (2010) G77(P) improving the recognition of domestic violence in an urban emergency department. Assoc Paediatr Emerg Med 100:A32

Valpied J, Hegarty K (2015) Intimate partner abuse: identifying, caring for and helping women in healthcare settings. Womens Health 11(1):51–63

von Eye A, Bogat GA (2006) Mental health in women experiencing intimate partner violence as the efficiency goal of social welfare functions. Int J Soc Welf 15:S31–S40

Wadman MC, Muelleman RL (1999) Domestic violence homicides: ED use before victimization. Am J Emerg Med 17:689–691

WHO (2010) Expert meeting on health-sector responses to violence against women. https://apps.who.int/iris/bitstream/handle/10665/44456/9789241500630_eng.pdf;sequence=1

WHO (2017) Violence against women: key facts. http://www.who.int/en/news-room/fact-sheets/detail/violence-against-women. Accessed 12 Apr 2019

Williston CJ, Lafreniere K (2013) 'Holy cow does that ever open up a can of worms': health care providers' experiences of inquiring about intimate partner violence. Health Care Women Int 34(9):814–831

WMA (2010) WMA statement on family violence. https://www.wma.net/wp-content/uploads/2017/02/Family_Violence-Oct2010.pdf. Accessed 12 Apr 2019

Yam M (2000) Seen but not heard: battered women's perceptions of the ED experience. J Emerg Nurs 26(5):464–470

Yeung H, Chowdhury N, Malpass A, Feder GS (2012) Responding to domestic violence in general practice: a qualitative study on perceptions and experiences. Int J Family Med 2012:960523. https://doi.org/10.1155/2012/960523

Barriers and Opportunities to Effective Identification and Management of Domestic Violence and Abuse

5

Kathryn Hinsliff-Smith

5.1 Introduction

As a healthcare professional, either as a qualified practitioner or as a student we are governed by the requirements of our own healthcare profession. You may work within a private or public funded clinical setting or employed in the voluntary sector working, for example, for a charity or hospice provider. Wherever you are an employed it is incumbent on you, as a healthcare professional across any spectrum of the profession to provide care for your patients. Your healthcare facility, in any country, is often uniquely placed and can play an essential role in responding, supporting and referring patients to appropriate services who have experienced domestic violence or abuse (DVA). In the UK, for example, there are clear signposting and specialist services available to support survivors and also for perpetrator programmes. This is often in addition to the support that can be provided at the time of first contact with healthcare services. The aim of this chapter is to explore the debates and evidence surrounding DVA, routine enquiry and the support mechanisms that are in place to support those working in clinical practice.

In the UK it is estimated that the cost of providing NHS care as a result of DVA, which may include multiple interactions with healthcare professionals, repeat visits to clinical settings and ongoing healthcare need, was estimated in 2004 to be as high as £1.7 billion per year (Walby and Allen 2004). This estimated cost does not include mental health costs, estimated at an additional £176 million (Walby and Allen 2004). In 2008, these estimates were updated and showed a significant increase in terms of an aggregate cost that includes medical and social services, lost economic output and emotional costs, as £15.7 billion ($29.1 billion) (Walby 2009). The considerable cost of DVA is well known by policy makers or those working in

K. Hinsliff-Smith (✉)
De Montfort University, Leicester, UK
e-mail: Kathryn.Hinsliff-Smith@dmu.ac.uk

© Springer Nature Switzerland AG 2020
P. Ali, J. McGarry (eds.), *Domestic Violence in Health Contexts: A Guide for Healthcare Professions*, https://doi.org/10.1007/978-3-030-29361-1_5

front line health and social care services but can only be provided as an estimate due to the very nature of DVA. Often survivors will not disclose or may require health interventions on multiple occasions before seeking help, often links are not made to undying medical conditions so the true costs for longer term healthcare needs are difficult to quantify, for example the effect of DVA on an individual's mental health and the subsequent need for ongoing support.

More broadly and in relation to DVA the World Health Organization (WHO) recommends the adoption of specialised training and education on DVA to try and stem the increasing numbers of those experiencing DVA (WHO 2017). The WHO also reports that one in three women (35%) across the world will experience some form of physical or sexual violence in their lifetime (Wyatt et al. 2019) and 38% of female murders globally are committed by an intimate partner (WHO 2017). As a consequence, this will undoubtedly directly impact upon the likelihood of health-care professionals, in any context and geographic region, required to provide care for survivors of DVA. Work conducted as far back as the early 1990s and before categorisation of DVA and the various types of abuse it was declared that:

> Abuse is a hidden health care problem, and the unsuspecting stance of health professionals allows the problem to remain undetected much of the time (Tilden et al. 1994: 632).

Within a UK context, for example, there are clear guidelines in place that indicate the management, support and referral pathways are the responsibility of health-care providers and there is a duty on any healthcare professional to be able to respond appropriately to their patients (NICE 2014, 2016). Further afield in the USA, for example, the U.S. Department of Health and Human Services, in their Healthy People 2010 policy, focussed on specific objectives to reduce the incidences of DVA (Davis and Harsh 2001). To try and address the need for recognition for DVA by healthcare professionals, the American Association of Colleges of Nurses (AACN) mandated that all pre-licensed (equivalent to UK registration) nurse education programmes should incorporate training on DVA (AACN 1999), although it is widely reported that this in itself has been slow to be fully integrated into the curriculum (Tufts et al. 2009). In other geographic regions, there are mixed responses to the need to train and educate healthcare professionals to recognise, respond and manage patients across any clinical settings. For example, within primary care in Kuwait there is a reported pressing need to provide national practice guidelines for DVA management that will provide the basis for clinicians to adhere and to be guided by (Alotaby et al. 2013) as currently these guidelines are reported as lacking. This is relevant to a range of healthcare professionals. For example, within the provision of midwifery, the Australia Department of Health provides clear guidelines for midwives and those in contact with families as a clinician's opportunity to identify, support and protect those at a vulnerable time (see Australian DoH). Within the UK, it is a requirement that all pregnant women will be routinely asked about their welfare and any safety concerns for them or their unborn child and this should be recorded in the women's health screening record.

What is widely evidenced is that survivors of DVA will call upon the services of healthcare professionals either at point of requiring immediate medical attention or as a result of experiencing some related medical condition. This may include, for example, acute or chronic conditions resulting from experiencing any form of DVA. Chronic conditions could be as broad as stress-related symptoms, mental health conditions, gastrointestinal symptoms or anxiety. What is often expressed by healthcare professionals who undertake any safeguarding training, which may include DVA training, is that patients may present what could be considered classic symptoms of a DVA-related incident. For example, portrayals of a broken arm, a bruised body or any other easily identifiable conditions that could immediately be linked to a case of DVA by an attending clinician (Alshammari et al. 2018).

What is difficult to accurately quantify is the prevalence of presentation as a result of DVA within any clinical setting. A recent systematic review (Hinsliff-Smith and McGarry 2017) explored what studies reported prevalence of DVA within ED settings as well as the reported management and support provided for patients who attended ED. With regard to prevalence it was widely accepted as a key dimension for recording incidents and is reliant on survivors disclosing at the time of presentation (Boyle et al. 2010). The literature is clear that survivors will not routinely report DVA but are more likely to disclose when clinician enquires (Evans et al. 2016; Mills et al. 2006) and this clinical interaction may result in seeing less repeat visits to the ED (Boyle et al. 2010). What is abundantly clear is that there is still no conclusive means to record incidents of DVA within any clinical settings or indeed a standardised mechanism in many countries. This is despite the acceptance that DVA is a major health concern and is cited as a 'pandemic' (Wyatt et al. 2019). The UK National Institute for Health and Care Excellence (NICE) guidelines (2014) are broadly welcomed as a means to address some of the concerns and challenges of supporting individuals and families who experience DVA as well as provide guidelines for the organisational structures and cultures to exist within our clinical settings (McGarry and Nairn 2015). This latter point directly relates to the means by which healthcare professionals, across any setting, are able to access the appropriate training and have the knowledge to provide the most appropriate care for their patients.

The systematic review conducted by Hinsliff-Smith and McGarry (2017) explored the management and support provided for DV in ED settings. The review reported that whilst the physical consequences of DVA were much easier to identify the emotional and psychological effects of DVA on survivors were often missed (Hinsliff-Smith and McGarry 2017) and concurs with work by Kramer et al. (2004). It was also reported that ED staff often lacked the knowledge and sufficient training to appropriately identify, manage and support survivors of DVA (Saberi et al. 2017; Robinson 2010).

For those working in front line services, like ED, as a healthcare professional you are often placed in a position whereby you want to provide medical care for your patient whilst develop trust and understanding with your patient in a short space of time, often against a backdrop of time pressures to move your patient along (Taylor et al. 2013). This is particularly telling where a time frame is applied to patient care, such as witnessed in the UK. A four hour target to see, treat and admit or discharge was introduced by the Department of Health in England in 2004 and is closely monitored for any breaching with financial penalties applied. Such a time frame requires that clinicians providing medical attention, and all that this may entail, at the same time as providing support and directing a patient to appropriate referral pathways if there is a disclosure or suspicion of DVA. Moreover, there is extensive literature that describes barriers that exist within these clinical settings. EDs are open 24/7 and are busy environments, receiving patients via ambulances as well as freely accessible for walk in patients. All will be requiring access to medical care for a multitude of conditions; some classed as accident and emergency cases. For patients this can be a scary and unfamiliar place which may be compounded by the fact that they have received injuries or experiencing conditions brought about from a DVA incident. However, evidence informs us that ED is often the very first point of contact for those who have experienced any injury resulting from DVA (Hinsliff-Smith and McGarry 2017; Rhodes et al. 2007; Yonaka et al. 2007). This is often the setting whereby the patient is likely to disclose to a clinician when asked appropriately or where a clinician is able to identify what might appear to be injuries related to DVA.

In addition to these reported barriers, it is also widely reported that providing staff with the necessary training and knowledge (Sprague et al. 2012; Sprague et al. 2017; Hoke et al. 2008) to identify, support and manage patients who have experienced DVA is essential (Wyatt et al. 2019; Ahmad et al. 2017; Alotaby et al. 2013; Ramsay et al. 2002, Davis and Harsh 2001). What is less clear is the type of training that is effective and in what settings, whether that be in the ED as advocated within the advocate model used within some ED departments in the UK (SafeLives 2015), or in primary care, a training programme aimed at GPs and staff working within general practice (IRIS model, see IRIS link), or a more holistic view that in order to provide comprehensive patient care state interventions are required (Alotaby et al. 2013).

Whilst this chapter is exploring the barriers and opportunities for the effective identification and management in relation to your clinical capacity, there is one further dimension to consider and that is the debate that surrounds whether we should routinely screen our patients for DVA.

As students or recently qualified healthcare professionals you may already have provided care for men, women or families who have experienced DVA. Indeed you may have been asked to complete a risk assessment form and submit a referral form for a patient. In the UK, there is a process whereby multiple agencies will review any submitted referral forms and meet to discuss any cases of DVA whereby the risk assessment score indicates a high or very high risk to the individual, children or family. A risk assessment score of seven or more will indicate a high or very high risk, those lower than seven could be categorised as 'standard' or 'medium' risk and could also be referred if there is a police concern. These meetings between multiple agencies are referred to as MARAC (Multi-Agency Risk Assessment Conferences) (Robbins et al. 2014). Whilst not all survivors will readily disclose an incident to a healthcare professional, indeed we are aware in the UK that women will experience up to 35 instances before they will seek support (SafeLives 2015) and that more than 20% of high-risk victims will attend ED as a result of their injuries in the year before they receive effective help (SafeLives 2015).

Let's focus on the ED for a moment. As mentioned earlier in this chapter, this is the clinical setting that we know more patients are likely to seek medical attention and may disclose or you suspect DVA as a cause. One argument for providing better targeted care and in turn providing the necessary support for survivors is to conduct *universal screening* of all patients. The nature of screening or 'routine enquiry' as it is sometimes referred to, put simply, means to use a proven method which asks patients to disclose if they have experienced any form of DVA which may relate to their current or past medical history. It is generally agreed that screening encompasses the use of set questions that are directly asked of all patients who attend for medical attention. Since ED is the most likely first point of contact for survivors and their families, then the debate predominately relates to routine screening within this clinical setting. Various approaches have been reported as to how to conduct screening, including computerised systems (Rhodes et al. 2006), paper based (Davis and Harsh 2001), surveys (Sethi et al. 2004; Boyle and Todd 2003; Kramer et al. 2004) and some later discussions about the framing of the questions (Evans et al. 2016) in the context that for many survivors there may be some difficulty in disclosing or articulating a DV incident (Feder et al. 2009).

Screening is not mandated across many healthcare services in different countries such as the USA or the UK and is still controversial and hotly debated (Hinsliff-Smith and McGarry 2017; Saberi et al. 2017; Devi 2012; Phelan 2007; Ramsay et al. 2002). Indeed, the arguments against universal screening are often cited against the safety of the survivor and children. In some states of the USA, for example, if a physician believed that a violent act has taken place, then they are required to report this to the police regardless if the victim agrees or not (Saberi et al. 2017). For many organisations involved in the safety of women there is obvious concern that this may endanger the lives of the survivor or stop any further disclosures from victims of DVA. There are also concerns that reporting the incident may lead to more harm and could escalate the abuse. This could then lead to survivors less inclined to disclose or report their perpetrators. In Canada, a large-scale study was conducted for testing out the use of screening and usual practice across 25 emergency departments, family practices or gynaecology clinics with 7000 female patients. They extensively reported that:

> These results do not provide sufficient evidence to support universal [domestic violence] screening in healthcare settings in the absence of an effective intervention to prevent or reduce abuse, especially in the context of the resources required to conduct screening and to deal with the number of women identified by the screening tool. (MacMillan et al. 2009)

A further dimension for introducing universal screening is the evidence from screening trials (Ahmad et al. 2017; Saberi et al. 2017; Davis and Harsh 2001) that indicate that by routinely screening the levels of detection for DVA are greatly increased. Contrary to that, a widely cited systematic review by Ramsay et al. (2002) also explored whether health professionals should screen women for DVA and found only ten sources from nine studies that explored routine screening

(Ramsay et al. 2002). Their overarching conclusions were that whilst routine screening did increase the detection rates and disclosure rates, there was no evidence of the long-term effects of routine screening. Therefore, based on the evidence they could not advocate for routine screening to be implemented in any clinical settings (Ramsay et al. 2002). This view concurs with the work by Anglin and Sachs (2003), who also conducted a review on screening tools and reported that there was no evidence for increasing rates of mortality or incidences from using screening.

Further work on this by Rhodes et al. (2006) who conducted a randomised control trial (RCT) for computer aided screening at two large EDs found that whilst disclosures increased there was still no guarantee of how the patient was supported or referred onwards to an appropriate pathway (Rhodes et al. 2006). This important aspect of identification and then supporting and managing the patient is fundamental if as clinicians, we are to reduce the incidences of DVA but also reduce the healthcare burden to the individuals as well as society. The work by Choo et al. (2012) in the USA on DVA screening also found that whilst resources were available for ED staff to support their patients after disclosure, injuries were not attributed to DVA and were often not noted in patient records. This lack of accurate recording will exasperate the ability to identify the true levels of DVA within any context and could lead to patient harm in the future.

The literature informs us that screening is purported to be an accepted method for EDs in the USA. For example, the most reported method for screening is the use of direct questions, either verbally or via a standard questionnaire administered to all patients (Phelan 2007) as a means to identify and assist with referral pathways or actions to protect them and their families if relevant. In the UK, we do not have routine enquiry or screening in any clinical setting, so we adopt an approach called *clinical enquiry* (RCN 2019). This is based on the principle that through your professional assessment of your patients if you suspect DVA you will use your clinical judgment to provide the necessary support and management for that patient. Likewise, when a patient confines in you that they have sustained injuries or have medical conditions related to DVA then you are required to provide the necessary support and advice about referral pathways. It has been argued that in order to identify and support patients who have experienced DVA then an overarching systems model approach (McCaw et al. 2001) needs to be adopted. Such a system would develop tools and resources for the effective support, referral and management of reporting DVA, support mechanisms for survivors, appropriate training for all frontline staff and networks established with organisations often outside of healthcare, such as social services, third sector organisations (often charities), the police, and primary/community care. In the UK, a randomised control trial (RCT) was conducted for testing usual care and an intervention involving the components described above (training, information, support and referral) as a systems approach model using GP practices as the clinical setting. The project, Identification, Referral to Improve Safety (IRIS) (see http://www.irisdomesticviolence.org.uk/iris/) study showed a significant difference between the intervention and usual care for the identification and management for survivors of DVA which has subsequently been commissioned and adopted across many UK GP practices (Feder et al. 2011). More recent work has also been undertaken within English EDs, maternity clinics and primary care whereby a trained advocate (IDVA) will be located in the clinical setting to provide support for staff and patients who require further advice or support at that time; this is often in addition to referral pathway advice (SafeLives 2015). In the UK, it is estimated that at least 1.2 million women and 784,000 men aged 16–59 have experienced some form of domestic violence and abuse in England and Wales in 2010/2011 (Osborne et al. 2012). Therefore, it is highly likely that during your professional clinical practice you may be required to provide care for a survivor of domestic violence, be a witness to DVA or be made aware of current or historical DVA by those that you work with. There is no recorded evidence for the prevalence of DVA as experienced by clinical staff who may have themselves experienced DVA and are expected to provide care for patients, but conversely there is evidence that this could be a factor and known barrier for staff to intervene (McGarry and Nairn 2015; Boyle and Todd 2006). In recognition that healthcare staff may themselves have experienced DVA, the National Health Service (NHS) provides guidance to support the creation and adoption of policies to support any NHS staff member. These are useful resources for you to explore (see NHS 2017).

In the UK, there are the NICE guidelines (2016, 2014) in addition to the professional body requirements to support and manage disclosures or suspicion of DVA. This may include gaining consent from a patient to escalate and therefore provide the patient with the necessary and appropriate support pathways that are available locally or nationally. In DVA instances that involve any family members under the age of 18, either as a witness to an incident (s) or directly in potential harm, then without the patient's consent it is your duty to record and report it to the appropriate authorities. This is the case whether there is a patient disclosure or suspicion of DVA. Each clinical area will have their own procedures in terms of escalation and it is incumbent upon you to locate and take the action to protect your patients and their families.

You should be aware that there are no typical survivors or perpetrators of DVA. It crosses all borders, nationalities, cultures and socioeconomic groupings and can affect men, women and children.

During your clinical training, DVA should be incorporated into any safeguarding training or indeed may be taught as a standalone module as is the case in many Higher Education Schools of Medicine or Allied Health Sciences programmes (Alshammari et al. 2018). Nothing can prepare you for the first encounter when your patient discloses or you witness what you feel to be injuries relating from a DVA incident, especially if your patient is not willing to confirm your suspicions. However, what we hope by reading the book is that it will enable you to be more aware of the magnitude and scale of DVA not just within the UK but wider as well as the different context that patients may present with DVA-related injuries and conditions. By reading this chapter we also hope that you can begin to understand the debate around routine screening and the alternative approach whereby clinical enquiry is advocated.

5.2   Summary

Our intention for providing this chapter in this groundbreaking book is for you, as the reader to consider your own position with regard to the use of routine screening or clinical enquiry as we have within the UK. Often when dealing with your patients, DV is often not black or white but often very complex and therefore requires you to develop a range of approaches and strategies not only to provide the very best clinical care but also to consider what your patient requires of you. You may also find that your clinical colleagues adopt different approaches and this can be for very different reasons. What is clear is that it is incumbent on you to follow the guidelines and policies in your own clinical area, not to judge your colleagues or indeed your patients, but to ensure that you have a consistent approach to the care provided for all your interactions with your patients.

Currently the view taken in many countries is that although DVA is a common problem with major health consequences for women, implementation of routine enquiry in healthcare settings cannot be justified (Ramsay et al. 2002). What is evident from the extant literature on DVA that has considered all aspects of care provided is the importance of engaging with healthcare professionals as well as including the voice of the care recipient, the DVA survivors. In doing so will help us to explore further the true benefits of specific DVA interventions in healthcare settings and if we were to have routine screening what are the implications of this for our patients, staff and the wider society.

Time to Reflect
Having read this chapter, we would now like you to review your own thoughts about routine screening compared to clinical enquiry for DVA.

Activity
Think about your current clinical placements or clinical workplace. How easy would it be for you to conduct a routine enquiry with your patients? What might be the barriers to conducting such an approach and how would you handle any disclosures? Would you know, for example, where and how to refer someone following disclosure of DVA?

Summary Points
• Having greater knowledge and awareness of the debate surrounding routine screening and clinical enquiry is necessary for practitioners.
• As a healthcare professional, you need to be aware of your own professional duty of care for your patients and how you might have to report any incidents without the patient's consent.
• Knowledge about screening may help you think about how to respond appropriately to disclosures and know how to refer and seek the appropriate pathway to support the survivor.

5.3   Web Resources

To extend your learning further about the aspects of DVA, we would encourage you to access these free online resources suitable for extending your knowledge about the subject of DVA. These are selections that are recommended:

1. Title: Gender Based Violence: a resource to support students in health and social care. https://www.nottingham.ac.uk/helmopen/rlos/safeguarding/gbv/index.html
2. Title: Safeguarding vulnerable people http://sonet.nottingham.ac.uk/rlos/placs/safeguarding/launcher.html
3. Title: Unlocking stories—Experiences of older women who are survivors of domestic violence and abuse https://www.nottingham.ac.uk/helmopen/rlos/safeguarding/unlocking-stories/
4. Unlocking the code https://www.nottingham.ac.uk/helmopen/rlos/unlocking-code/index.html
5. Silence to Voice: Co-design with survivors, students, academics digital resources on sexual violence in a South African context https://www.nottingham.ac.uk/toolkits/play_21204

References

Ahmad I, Ali PA, Rehman S, Talpur A, Dhingra K (2017) Intimate partner violence screening in emergency department: a rapid review of the literature. J Clin Nurs 26(21-22):3271–3285

Alotaby IY, Alkandari BA, Alshamali KA (2013) Barriers for domestic violence screening in primary health care centers. Alexandria J Med 49:175–180. https://doi.org/10.1016/j.ajme.2012.07.005

Alshammari KF, McGarry J, Higginbottom GMA (2018) Nurse education and understanding related to domestic violence and abuse against women: an integrative review of the literature. Nurs Open 5:237–253. https://doi.org/10.1002/nop2.133

American Association of Colleges and Nursing (AACN) (1999) Violence as a public health problem. https://www.aacnnursing.org/News-Information/Position-Statements-White-Papers/Violence-Problem. Accessed 5 May 2019

Anglin D, Sachs C (2003) Preventive care in the emergency department: screening for domestic violence in the emergency department. Acad Emerg Med 10(10):1118–1127

Australian Government Department of Health (n.d.). https://beta.health.gov.au/resources/pregnancy-care-guidelines/part-e-social-and-emotional-screening/family-violence. Accessed 3 Apr 2019

Boyle A, Todd C (2003) Incidence and prevalence of domestic violence in a UK emergency department. Emerg Med J 20(5):438–442

Boyle A, Todd C (2006) The acceptability of routine inquiry about domestic violence towards women: a survey in three healthcare settings. Br J Gen Pract 56:258–261

Boyle A, Frith C, Edgcumbe D, McDougall C (2010) What factors are associated with repeated domestic assault in patients attending an emergency department? A cohort study. Emerg Med J 27:203–206. https://doi.org/10.1136/emj.2009.072033

Choo E, Nicolaidis C, Newgard C, Lowe R, Hall M, McConnell K (2012) The association between emergency department resources and diagnosis of intimate partner violence. J Emerg Med 19(2):83–88. https://doi.org/10.1097/MEJ.0b013e328348a9f2

Davis RE, Harsh KE (2001) Confronting barriers to universal screening for domestic violence. J Prof Nurs 17(6):313–320. https://doi.org/10.1053/jpnu.2001.28181

Devi S (2012) US guidelines for domestic violence screening spark debate. Lancet 379(February):11. Accessed 12 Mar 2019

Evans M, Gregory A, Feder G, Howarth E, Hegarty K (2016) "Even 'daily' is not enough": how well do we measure domestic violence and abuse?—a think-aloud study of a commonly used self-report scale. Violence Vict 31(1):3–26. https://doi.org/10.1891/0886-6708.VV-D-15-00024

Feder G, Ramsay J, Dunne D, Rose M, Arsene C, Norman R (2009) How far does screening women for domestic (partner) violence in different health-care settings meet criteria for a screening programme? Systematic reviews of nine UK National Screening Committee criteria. Health Technol Assess 13(16):iii-iv, xi-xiii, 1–113, 137–347

Feder G, Davies RA, Baird K et al (2011) Identification and referral to improve safety (IRIS) of women experiencing domestic violence with a primary care training and support programme: a cluster randomised controlled trial. Lancet 378:1788–1795

Hinsliff-Smith K, McGarry J (2017) Understanding management and support for domestic violence and abuse within emergency departments: a systematic literature review from 2000–2015. J Clin Nurs 26(23-24):4013–4027

Hoke N (2008) Barriers to screening for domestic violence in the emergency department. J Trauma Nurs 15(2):79

Kramer A, Lorenzon D, Mueller G (2004) Prevalence of intimate partner violence and health implications for women using emergency departments and primary care clinics. Womens Health Issues 14:19–29. https://doi.org/10.1016/j.whi.2003.12.002

MacMillan HL, Wathen CN, Jamieson E et al (2009) Screening for intimate partner violence in health care settings—a randomized trial. JAMA 302(5):493–501. https://doi.org/10.1001/jama.2009.1089

McCaw B et al (2001) Beyond screening for domestic violence: a systems model approach in a managed care setting. Am J Prev Med 21(3):170–176. https://doi.org/10.1016/S0749-3797(01)00347-6

McGarry J, Nairn S (2015) An exploration of the perceptions of emergency department nursing staff towards the role of a domestic abuse nurse specialist: a qualitative study. Int Emerg Nurs 23(2):65–70. https://doi.org/10.1016/j.enj.2014.06.003

NHS (2017) Domestic violence and abuse: supporting NHS staff. https://www.nhsemployers.org/-/media/Employers/Publications/Health-and-wellbeing/HSWPG_DV_Policy-document.pdf

NICE (2014). https://www.nice.org.uk/guidance/qs116

NICE (2016) Domestic violence and abuse NICE quality standard [QS116]. National Institute of Clincial Excellence, London. https://www.nice.org.uk/guidance/qs116

Osborne S, Lau I, et al (2012) In: Smith K (ed) Homicides, firearm offences and intimate violence 2010/11: supplementary volume 2 to crime in England and Wales 2010/11. Home Office, London

Phelan M (2007) Screening for intimate partner violence in medical settings. Trauma Violence Abuse 8(2):199–213. https://doi.org/10.1177/1524838007301221. Accessed 2 Mar 2019

Ramsay J, Richardson J, Carter YH, Davidson L, Feder G (2002) Should health professionals screen women for domestic violence? Systematic review. BMJ 325(7359):314

RCN (2019). https://www.rcn.org.uk/clinical-topics/domestic-violence-and-abuse/national-guidance. Accessed 5 Apr 2019

Rhodes K, Drum M, Anliker E, Frankel R, Howes D, Levinson W (2006) Lowering the threshold for discussions of domestic violence: a randomized controlled trial of computer screening. Arch Intern Med 166:1107–1114. https://doi.org/10.1001/archinte.166.10.1107

Rhodes K, Frankel R, Levinthal N, Prenoveau E, Bailey J, Levinson W (2007) "You're not a victim of domestic violence, are you?" provider-patient communication about domestic violence. Ann Intern Med 147:620–627. https://doi.org/10.7326/0003-4819-147-9-200711060-00006

Robbins R, McLaughlin H, Banks C, Bellamy C, Thackray D (2014) Domestic violence and multi-agency risk assessment conferences (MARACs): a scoping review. J Adult Protect 16(6):389–398, 1466-8203. https://doi.org/10.1108/JAP-03-2014-0012

Robinson R (2010) Myths and stereotypes: how registered nurses screen for intimate partner violence. J Emerg Nurs 36(6):572–576. https://doi.org/10.1016/j.jen.2009.09.008

Saberi E et al (2017) Ready, willing and able? A survey of clinicians' perceptions about domestic violence screening in a regional hospital emergency department. Australas Emerg Nurs J 20(2):82–86

SafeLives (2015) Insights Idva national dataset 2013–14. SafeLives, Bristol

SafeLives (2016) A cry for health why we must invest in domestic abuse services in hospitals. Themis. http://www.safelives.org.uk/sites/default/files/resources/SAFJ4993_Themis_report_WEBcorrect.pdf. Accessed 12 Mar 2019

SafeLives (n.d.). http://www.safelives.org.uk/policy-evidence/about-domestic-abuse/how-long-do-people-live-domestic-abuse-and-when-do-they-get. Accessed 1 May 2019

Sethi D, Watts S, Zwi A, Watson J, McCarthy C (2004) Experience of domestic violence by women attending an inner city accident and emergency department. Emerg Med J 21(2):180–184

Sprague S, Madden K, Simunovic N, Godin K, Pham NK, Bhandari M, Goslings JC (2012) Barriers to screening for intimate partner violence. Women Health 52(6):587–605

Sprague S, Scott T, Garibaldi A et al (2017) A scoping review of intimate partner violence assistance programmes within health care settings. Eur J Psychotraumatol 8:1314159. https://doi.org/10.1080/20008198.2017.1314159

Taylor J, Bradbury-Jones C, Kroll T, Duncan F (2013) Health professionals' beliefs about domestic abuse and the issue of disclosure: a critical incident technique study. Health Soc Care Community 21(5):489–499

Tilden V, Schmidt T, Limandri B, Chiodo G, Garland M, Loveless P (1994) Factors that influence clinicians assessment and management of family violence. Am J Public Health 84:928–633

Tufts KA, Clements PT, Karlowicz KA (2009) Integrating intimate partner violence content across curricula: developing a new generation of nurse educators. Nurse Educ Today 29:40–47. https://doi.org/10.1016/j.nedt.2008.06.005

Walby S (2009). The cost of domestic violence: up-date 2009. United Nations educational, scientific and cultural organization. Lancaster University, Lancaster

Walby S, Allen J (2004) Domestic violence, sexual assault and stalking: finding from the British Crime Survey. Home Office Research Study 276. Home Office, London

WHO (2017) Violence against women. https://www.who.int/news-room/fact-sheets/detail/violence-against-women. Accessed 5 Nov 2019

Wyatt T, McClelland ML, Spangaro J (2019) Readiness of newly licensed associated degree registered nurses to screen for domestic violence. Nurse Edu Pract 35:75–82

Yonaka L, Yoder M, Darrow J, Sherck J (2007) Barriers to screening for domestic violence in the emergency department. J Contin Educ Nurs 38(1):37–45. PMID: 17269438

Domestic Violence and Abuse and Children: Principles of Practitioner Responses

6

Caroline Bradbury-Jones, Anita Morris, Dana Sammut, and Cathy Humphreys

6.1 Introduction

In the domestic violence and abuse (DVA) literature, it is only relatively recently that the impacts on children have been fully recognised, documented and researched. In this chapter, we explore the key issues for children and we emphasise the importance of ensuring that they are always considered in cases of suspected or known DVA. The chapter is loosely structured around a framework that two of the authors (Humphreys and Bradbury-Jones) proposed in 2015 as a way to help healthcare professionals support families and children affected by DVA through keeping in mind three domains: focus, response and intervention (Humphreys and Bradbury-Jones 2015).

Statistics relating to the prevalence of children's exposure to DVA can vary widely, depending on variables such as the definition of abuse, the time frame being described and the study sample. However, it is estimated that one in five children in the UK, and one in four in Australia have experienced DVA by 18 years of age (Radford et al. 2011; Indermaur 2001). Globally, estimates suggest that between 133 and 275 million children are exposed to DVA each year (UNICEF and The Body Shop International 2006). Children's experiences range from directly experiencing child abuse themselves, being hurt when intervening, to witnessing the violence or hearing events from afar. Their childhood may be marred by growing up in an atmosphere of fear (Stanley 2011), where there is threatened stability within the home and undermining of relationships between mothers, fathers and children (Laing et al. 2013). As we discuss in the following section, DVA has a serious, negative impact on the lives of children.

C. Bradbury-Jones (✉) · D. Sammut
University of Birmingham, Birmingham, UK
e-mail: c.bradbury-jones@bham.ac.uk

A. Morris · C. Humphreys
University of Melbourne, Melbourne, VIC, Australia

© Springer Nature Switzerland AG 2020
P. Ali, J. McGarry (eds.), *Domestic Violence in Health Contexts: A Guide for Healthcare Professions*, https://doi.org/10.1007/978-3-030-29361-1_6

6.2   Impacts of Domestic Violence on Health and Wellbeing

Coordinated Action Against Domestic Abuse (CAADA) (2014) (now Safe Lives) reported that children living with DVA suffered multiple physical and mental health consequences as a result: over half (52%) had behavioural problems, over a third (39%) had difficulties adjusting at school and nearly two-thirds (60%) felt responsible or to blame for negative events. For children who live in homes where DVA is occurring, the violence may be normalised as a way of resolving conflict (Blair et al. 2015). The effects are not the same between girls and boys, which leads to different risk factors for perpetration (boys) and victimisation (girls) in their own intimate relationships (Gover et al. 2008; Whitfield et al. 2003), thus reflecting the intergenerational aspects of DVA. While care needs to be taken to reassure children and young people that their adult lives can be different from their childhood, there are some gendered patterns that emerge in the data. Boys are significantly more likely to display externalising behaviour such as aggression and hostility, with potential influence on their own future intimate relationships. For young women though, intimate partner abuse in their own relationships can be part of a more complex picture, exposing them to other vulnerabilities including: going missing, sexual exploitation, forced marriage, teenage pregnancy, self-harm, substance misuse and gang involvement.

There are a number of other factors to consider in the discussion of intimate partner abuse among adolescents. For example, a study by Smith et al. (2003) found that young women who experience dating violence or abuse between the ages of 14–18 are statistically more likely to be physically or sexually 'revictimised' as young adults. Furthermore, a research synthesis by Stonard et al. (2014) highlights the emerging role of technology as an avenue for abuse among adolescents in romantic relationships. One example is the practice of 'sexting', which is defined as 'the creating, sharing and forwarding of sexually suggestive nude or nearly nude images' via mobile phones or the internet (Lenhart 2009: 3). While this practice is not unique to adolescents, a report by Ringrose et al. (2012) concludes that sexting among young people is often coercive, with girls in particular being vulnerable to denigration by their peers. The role of technology is a relatively new area of interest in the literature on adolescent dating violence, although it is likely to garner increasing attention as the impact, and use of online social network platforms continues to grow.

It also needs to be recognised that not all children are equally affected by DVA. Children and young people live in different contexts of vulnerability and protection. In any sample, there will be approximately a third of children who at a particular point in time appear to be doing as well as other children in the community (Kitzmann et al. 2003; Humphreys et al. 2018, 2019). Children have a right to live in nonabusive environments, but not all children will need the same response based on an assessment of their resilience and the protective factors that may surround them.

Table 6.1 Focus, response and intervention for children in the context of domestic violence

Focus	
1.	Foreground the voices and concerns of women and their children
2.	Recognise that there is both a child victim and an adult victim (usually, but not always, the child's mother)
3.	View DVA as an attack on the mother–child relationship
4.	Keep the perpetrator in view
Response	
5.	Consider separation as a time of heightened risk for lethality and severe abuse
6.	Respond to DVA within complex cases as a priority (where there is co-occurrence of domestic abuse, mental health and drug and alcohol problems)
Intervention	
7.	Target risk assessment and risk management on the perpetrator of DVA whilst providing support to remain safe to child and adult victims

Adapted from Humphreys and Bradbury-Jones (2015)

6.3   Current Good Practice and Evidence

The intergenerational effects of experiencing DVA can begin to occur as early as in utero and continue throughout the lifespan, demonstrating the need for practice approaches that identify early and respond accordingly (Ludy-Dobson and Perry 2010; Lieberman 2007). In this section, we turn our attention to what can be done to support children and families when DVA is a feature of their lives. The framework for safeguarding children in the context of DVA is explored further through the three key areas mentioned earlier: focus, response and intervention (Humphreys and Bradbury-Jones 2015). These are detailed in Table 6.1.

Time to Reflect
Table 6.1 shows how foregrounding the voices and concerns of women and children is essential. What do you think this means? How might it be achieved?
   It might be useful to talk through your responses with a colleague or friend.

6.4   Focus

There is a wealth of evidence suggesting that DVA is an under-reported problem (European Union Agency for Fundamental Rights 2014; O'Doherty et al. 2015). This, coupled with the fact that many healthcare professionals lack confidence in their ability to adequately respond to abuse disclosure (Sprague et al. 2012), means that many women and their children will not receive the support they need. There are a number of reasons why women might feel reluctant to disclose abuse, including fears that their abuser will find out, concerns about legal repercussions and even feelings of shame (Feder et al. 2009). However, research suggests that women are generally comfortable for the subject of DVA to be raised by their care providers, regardless of whether or not they choose to disclose abuse (Koziol-McLain et al. 2008; Spangaro et al. 2011).

Barriers to disclosure also exist from the healthcare professional's point-of-view. A qualitative focus group study by Spangaro et al. (2011) found that care providers are often worried about a potential conflict between their desire to maintain confidentiality and duty to escalate concerns to other agencies. Other research suggests that professionals are worried that they will offend or 'retraumatise' women by enquiring about abuse (Aluko et al. 2015). These issues can perhaps be alleviated, to an extent, in settings where patients and clients are able to build a relationship of trust over time with their care providers (for example, midwifery services in antenatal settings). However, the problem of healthcare professionals' lack of confidence in this area is arguably the biggest barrier to encouraging disclosure of abuse.

When considering how healthcare professionals can respond to young people experiencing DVA, Houghton (2015) explored the ethics of working with young people and suggested that young people provide a sensitised understanding of the relationship between their own safety and well-being and that of their mothers. Houghton (2015) shows how encouragement and supportive action can assist young people in being powerful political advocates for other young people and their mothers. She proposes that there are three E's of young people's participation in their own lives and decision-making: enjoyment, empowerment and emancipation. It is useful here to consider whether these three issues came into your responses to reflective activity 1.

Maternal protectiveness in the context of DVA is a complex issue and Nicola Moulding et al. (2015) untangle the complexity of strengthening relationships between mothers and children on one hand, while simultaneously safeguarding children on the other. They describe this as a careful balancing act that is nevertheless a crucial part of practice for those who work with DVA. Their study highlighted the dynamic of self-blame among mothers, and mother-blame among adults who were exposed to DVA in childhood. That is why in Table 6.1, we highlight the impacts of DVA on both mother and child and importantly, how the relationship between them can be fractured (but also strengthened or recovered).

An important part of the focus is to understand the strategies of coercive control that were used by the perpetrator of violence, to understand their impact and the harm that was done to the child, the mother–child relationship, and the ecology of the family (Humphreys et al. 2018; Humphreys et al. 2019). Such is the enduring omnipresence of perpetrators, that women are often left questioning whether he is an 'absent presence' or in fact more present than absent in the child's life (Thiara and Humphreys 2017; Humphreys et al. 2018, 2019). Hence the need to keep the perpetrator 'in view', as per Table 6.1.

6.5   Response

Children need to know their fathers but a meaningful relationship is not possible when abuse to either the child or the child's mother continues. Children have a right to leave an abusive relationship and it is not a matter of choice, but rather, a right that needs to be honoured by all decision-makers and particularly the courts (Humphreys and Bradbury-Jones 2015). What needs to be considered though, are the considerable risks and 'lethality' faced by women and children in the post-separation period. A profound shortcoming of the safeguarding response lies in under-estimating the ongoing harm to children in the post-separation period. This is reflected in Table 6.1, which highlights the complexities of DVA particularly in relation to other issues including drugs and alcohol, and crucially, the 'heightened risk of lethality' and ongoing abuse that can occur following separation (Campbell et al. 2003).

In a qualitative study, Fiona Morrison (2015) conducted in-depth interviews with children (aged 8–14) and their mothers to explore the outcomes of post-separation contact arrangements between the children and their fathers. A key finding of the study was that the end of a relationship does *not* mark the end of abuse. In fact, during the period immediately following separation, many women reported an escalation of abusive behaviour from their ex-partners, with several women commenting that they feared for their lives. Some children also reported experiencing abuse themselves during organised contact with their fathers, ranging from emotional to physical. Beyond this, many children had to make difficult decisions when trying to bridge the communication gap between their parents. Morrison concludes by arguing that 'abusive men need to be held accountable for their behaviour *before* contact begins' (p. 283).

Anna Nikupeteri et al. (2015) explored children's experiences of post-separation stalking by their fathers. Citing earlier studies (Mechanic et al. 2000; Sheridan and Roberts 2011), the authors noted that stalking that occurs following abusive intimate relationships tends to be more physically violent than stranger stalking, or stalking following *non-abusive* intimate relationships. Their study describes three 'forms' of children's security which emerge in response to paternal stalking: eroded (where children begin to lose trust in their father, despite believing that he cannot truly hurt them), lost (realising that the threat of violence is real) and reconstructed (taking steps to safeguard themselves, their mother and siblings). This research demonstrates the impact on children of paternal stalking, and highlights the very real risk of escalated violence during the post-separation period, offering a counter to the rhetoric of 'If it was that bad, she'd leave him'.

More recent research and practice reiterates that there may have been an inappropriate conflation of separation and safety (Holt 2015). Women and children made homeless, or their residency status lost, or long periods of unsupervised access with fathers who use violence belie the safety of separation. Strenuous efforts may need to be made to focus on the father who uses violence and whether he has any capacity and interest in changing his behaviour (Stanley and Humphreys 2017).

> **Case Study 1 Domestic Violence: Focus and Response in Health Settings**
> Jane often attends the local health clinic with her children, Peter, 12 years old, and Mara who is 8 years old. The visits focus on the children's common ailments, however the general practitioner (GP) has recognised that Jane is struggling emotionally, and her physical health appears to have declined. The GP invites Jane to make an appointment to see him on her own next visit so he can focus on her health needs and also ask sensitively about DVA as he is aware of difficulties in Jane's relationship with her partner.

At the next visit Jane attends alone and guided by the GP's gentle questioning about Jane's relationship and feelings of fear towards her partner, Jane feels safe to disclose that her partner Paul is in fact perpetrating DVA—physical, emotional and sexual violence.

The GP listens and validates her experience. He pre-empts the need to be alert to the possibility of child abuse and neglect and explains to Jane that he will work with her to understand the risks her partner may pose to her and the children and use the opportunity to think about safety planning for the family. He offers to link her to services and suggests a follow-up visit for Jane to attend with the children. They negotiate that Jane will raise at the next visit that there are arguments occurring at home and that this is having an impact on everyone. Peter and Mara will each be given an opportunity to respond to this comment and Jane will help them to feel comfortable to disclose what this is like for each of them. The GP will listen to each child, talk with them directly and validate their experience. He will discuss supports available to the children (whether they disclose any issues or not) such as school, counselling, and other opportunities for mentoring and support. Jane and the GP will model the ability to talk about the violence occurring in the home in a safe way that supports help-seeking. The GP will of course be alert to the need for a statutory response and be proactive in talking about the types of services that can work with families in the event that children are unsafe. Follow-up visits are arranged to enable review of risk, safety planning, and engagement or otherwise with services.

Time to Reflect
Read Case Study 1 that describes the situation of Jane and her two children Peter and Mara.
Make some notes on how you think the actions of Jane's GP meet the focus and response requirements that we outline in Table 6.1.
Make a list of what you think might be the barriers to the GP's effective response and support of Jane and her children.
What are the barriers to communication and disclosure that Jane may be experiencing?

6.6 Intervention

Safeguarding children and young people living with DVA has emerged as a priority area across health, justice and human service sectors. The past few decades have seen a gradual shift in ideology, practice and service organisation in relation to DVA (Humphreys and Bradbury-Jones 2015). Responding to the needs of children and families living with DVA has shifted from an issue of concern only for women's DVA organisations into one involving mainstream organisations (Walby et al. 2014). Mainstreaming is associated with infusion of ideas developed within the specialist DVA sector into organisations such as police, child protection and courts and growing awareness within the generalist and universal services such as hospitals, schools and early childhood centres of the need and opportunity to recognise family violence and intervene earlier.

A suite of different developments have now occurred which focus on strengthening the mother–child relationship in the aftermath of violence (Humphreys et al. 2015). Some of the stronger evidence comes from randomised control trials conducted in the USA (Lieberman et al. 2006), though there are many other programs working with mother–child dyads such as Mothers in Mind (Jenney and Sura-Liddell 2008) or parallel groups for women and children (Graham-Bermann et al. 2007). Smith et al. (2015) report on the evaluation of an intervention called 'Domestic Abuse Recovering Together' (DART). The 10-week DART programme focuses on rebuilding a threatened and undermined mother–child relationship after abuse. The study showed promising results, demonstrating increased levels of affection from mothers to their children following the programme. The paper provides an important anti-deterministic message: although domestic abuse can have a detrimental effect on the mother–child relationship, intervention programmes can be effective (Smith et al. 2015).

In the land of evidence-based policy what counts as 'success' or 'what works' becomes critical to commissioners of services (Humphreys and Bradbury-Jones 2015). Howarth et al. (2015) draw attention to the incongruity between children's and their mothers' perspectives on 'success', and those outcome measures used in research evaluation. Howarth et al.'s (2015) paper raises important concerns about the ways in which there may be a disconnection between programme outcome measures (e.g. mental health and behavioural issues) and the issues that children and their mothers prioritise in healing and recovery. The paper reinforces the need for voices of women and children to be taken seriously (Howarth et al. 2015).

A recent synthesis of qualitative research into children's own perspectives on their experiences of DVA emphasised the need for professionals to take account of the range of children's experiences and the need to listen intently to each child's own narrative (Arai et al. 2019). Assumptions are often made about children's 'best interests' without attention to the ways in which they may voice or act out their concerns. An intervention 'for' children rather than 'with' children has often been a basic flaw in the intervention that will continually need to be addressed. Participatory methods including co-design of policy and practice interventions have the potential to address this issue from the outset and have begun to be used successfully in DVA research and programme development with adults via experience-led co-design (Tarzia et al. 2017).

6.7   Reflection and Identification of Further Learning

Box 6.1 Dealing with Domestic Violence in Practice: Crucial Conversations
Patterson et al. (2012) refer to 'crucial conversations' as those that may contain: (1) opposing opinions (2) strong emotions and/or (3) high stakes. 'Crucial conversations' are vital in opening up discussions about DVA with children and families and providing opportunity for disclosure (Bradbury-Jones 2015).

This can break cycles of silence and provide opportunities for safety planning. Talking sensitively and directly to the child may create opportunities for a disclosure. Some children do not want to talk, others disclose indirectly or disclose in a roundabout way, for example: '*Sometimes my stepdad upsets my mum*'. The child is hoping that someone will pick up on the indirect message about their experiences. Ask simple questions, such as: '*Is there something you're sad or worried about?*'

The Ministry of Health New Zealand guidelines (Fanslow et al. 2016) suggest some helpful validation statements that reflect sentiments such as: '*I believe you, I am glad you came to me, I am sorry this has happened, You're not to blame, We are going to do something together to get help*'.

In all events, it is crucial that you don't wait until you are certain about what is happening in a child's life before responding to your concerns regarding a child's experience of DVA.

6.8 Summary

This chapter has reiterated the importance of understanding children as victims of DVA in their own right. Taking this lead, legislative definitions of DVA in the UK and Australia now include reference to children's exposure. The negative impacts of family violence on children are now well documented in the literature. These impacts can occur very early in life and continue into adolescence and adulthood. The concept of intergenerational transmission of DVA has been used to describe how DVA can impact children who then go on to experience either victimisation or perpetration of violence in their own intimate relationships.

Through the framework proposed previously by Humphreys and Bradbury-Jones (2015)—focus, response and intervention—professionals are supported in their safeguarding of children. The framework pertains to the familial triad which includes: individual and shared issues; opportunities for mother and child strengthening, and recognition of the perpetrator's impact on this relationship. The framework outlines increased risk associated with separation, and the importance of prioritising DVA cases that feature compounding factors such as mental health and drug and alcohol problems, whilst focusing risk assessment and management on perpetrator behaviour and victim safety and support.

Healthcare professionals' recognition of children's need for enjoyment, empowerment and emancipation sits alongside the need to safeguard the child and strengthen the mother–child relationship. There is the need for a deep understanding of how a perpetrator undermines the mother–child relationship that has repercussions for the bond into adolescence and beyond.

No longer can we ignore the voices of children and young people experiencing DVA. Through crucial conversations, healthcare professionals have the tools to listen, validate and support children, young people and their mothers for safer outcomes.

Summary Points

- Children can be exposed to DVA in a number of ways, both directly and indirectly. This exposure is known to have serious and lasting negative impacts, with many children going on to experience violence in their adolescent and adult intimate relationships.
- The voices of children and women must remain a central focus in all crucial conversations. Patterns of abusive behaviour are not always immediately obvious—for example, in cases of coercive control—and so the perpetrator must always be kept 'in view' by healthcare professionals.
- Violence often escalates during the post-separation period. It is important for professionals to realise that separation does not equate to safety, and ongoing support for children and their mothers will be required after the event.
- Many healthcare professionals lack the knowledge and confidence required to respond to DVA effectively. Familiarisation with the three key areas of focus, response and intervention will encourage a safe and evidence-based approach to addressing this complex issue in practice.

References

Aluko OE, Beck KH, Howard DE (2015) Medical students' beliefs about screening for intimate partner violence: a qualitative study. Health Promot Pract 16(4):540–549

Arai L, Heawood A, Feder G, Howarth E, MacMillan H, Moore THM et al (2019) Hope, agency, and the lived experience of violence: a qualitative systematic review of children's perspectives on domestic violence and abuse. Trauma Violence Abuse. https://doi.org/10.1177/1524838019849582

Blair F, McFarlane J, Nava A, Gilroy H, Maddoux J (2015) Child witness to domestic abuse: baseline data analysis for a seven-year prospective study. Pediatr Nurs 41(1):23–29

Bradbury-Jones C (2015) Talking about domestic abuse: crucial conversations for health visitors. Community Pract 88(12):44–47

Campbell JC, Webster D, Koziol-McLain J, Block C, Campbell D, Curry A et al (2003) Risk factors for femicide in abusive relationships: results from a multisite case control study. Am J Public Health 93:1089–1097

Co-ordinated Action Against Domestic Abuse (CAADA) (2014) In plain sight: the evidence from children exposed to domestic abuse. http://www.safelives.org.uk/sites/default/files/resources/In_plain_sight_the_evidence_from_children_exposed_to_domestic_abuse.pdf

European Union Agency for Fundamental Rights (2014) Violence against women: an EU-wide survey, European Union agency for fundamental rights. https://fra.europa.eu/en/publication/2014/violence-against-women-eu-wide-survey-main-results-report. Accessed 6 May 2019

Fanslow JL, Kelly P, Ministry of Health (2016) Family violence assessment and intervention guideline: child abuse and intimate partner violence, 2nd edn. Ministry of Health, Wellington

Feder G, Ramsay J, Dunne D, Rose M, Arsene C, Norman R, Kuntze S, Spencer A, Bacchus L, Hague G, Warburton A, Taket A (2009) How far does screening women for domestic (partner) violence in different health-care settings meet criteria for a screening programme? Systematic reviews of nine UK National Screening Committee criteria. Health Technol Assess 13:1–1136

Gover AR, Kaukinen C, Fox KA (2008) The relationship between violence in the family of origin and dating violence among college students. J Interpers Violence 23(12):1667–1693

Graham-Bermann SA, Lynch S, Banyard V, DeVoe ER, Halabu H (2007) Community-based intervention for children exposed to intimate partner violence: an efficacy trial. J Consult Clin Psychol 75(2):199

Holt S (2015) Post-separation fathering and domestic abuse: challenges and contradictions. Child Abuse Rev 24(3):210–222

Houghton C (2015) Young people's perspectives on a participatory ethics: agency, power and impact in domestic abuse research and policy-making. Child Abuse Rev 24:235–248

Howarth E, Moore T, Heawood A, Hester M, MacMillan H, Stanley N, Welton N, Feder G (2015) Measuring the effectiveness of targeted interventions for children exposed to domestic violence: measuring success in ways that matter to children and parents. Child Abuse Rev 24:231–234

Humphreys C, Bradbury-Jones C (2015) Domestic abuse and safeguarding: focus, response and intervention. Child Abuse Rev 24(4):231–234

Humphreys C, Thiara RK, Sharp C, Jones J (2015) Supporting the relationship between mothers and children in the aftermath of domestic violence. In: Stanley N, Humphreys C (eds) Domestic violence and child protection: new challenges and developments. Jessica Kingsley Publications, London, pp 130–147

Humphreys C, Healey L, Nicholson D, Kirkwood D (2018) Making the case for a differential child protection response for children living with domestic and family violence. Aust Soc Work 71:162–174

Humphreys C, Diemer K, Bornemisza A, Spiteri-Staines A, Kaspiew R, Horsfall B (2019) More present than absent: men who use domestic violence and their fathering. Child Fam Soc Work 24:321–329. https://doi.org/10.1111/cfs.12617

Indermaur D (2001) Young Australians and domestic violence. Trends and issues in crime and criminal justice no. 195. Issues paper. Australian Institute of Criminology, Canberra

Jenney A, Sura-Liddell L (2008) Mothers in mind: an attachment informed intervention for abused women with infants and toddlers'. Paper presented at The Hospital for Sick Children, Toronto, Canada

Kitzmann KM, Gaylord NK, Holt AR, Kenny ED (2003) Child witnesses to domestic violence: a meta-analytic review. J Consult Clin Psychol 71(2):339

Koziol-McLain J, Giddings L, Rameka M, Fyfe E (2008) Intimate partner violence screening and brief intervention: experiences of women in two New Zealand health care settings. J Midwifery Womens Health 53:504–510

Laing L, Humphreys C, Cavanagh K (2013) Social work and domestic violence: critical and reflective practice. Sage Publications, London

Lenhart A (2009) Teens and sexting: how and why minor teens are sending sexually suggestive nude or nearly nude images via text messaging. Pew Research Centre Report. https://www.pewinternet.org/2009/12/15/teens-and-sexting/. Accessed 20 June 2019

Lieberman AF (2007) Ghosts and angels: intergenerational patterns in the transmission and treatment of the traumatic sequelae of domestic violence. Infant Ment Health J 28(4):422–439

Lieberman AF, Ghosh Ippen C, Van Horn P (2006) Child-parent psychotherapy: 6-month follow-up of a randomized controlled trial. J Am Acad Child Adolesc Psychiatry 45(8):913–918

Ludy-Dobson CR, Perry BD (2010) The role of healthy relational interactions in buffering the impact of childhood trauma. Working with children to heal interpersonal trauma: the power of play. pp. 26–43

Mechanic M, Weaver T, Resick P (2000) Intimate partner violence and stalking behavior: exploration of patterns and correlations in a sample of acutely battered women. Violence Vict 15:55–72

Morrison F (2015) 'All over now?' The ongoing relational consequences of domestic abuse through children's contact arrangements. Child Abuse Rev 24:274–284

Moulding N, Buchanan F, Wendt S (2015) Untangling self-blame and mother-blame in women's and children's perspectives on maternal protectiveness in domestic violence: implications for practice. Child Abuse Rev 24:249–260

Nikupeteri A, Tervonen H, Laitinen M (2015) Eroded, lost or reconstructed? Security in Finnish Children's experiences of post-separation stalking. Child Abuse Rev 24:285–296

O'Doherty L, Hegarty K, Ramsay J, Davison L, Feder G Taft A (2015) Screening women for intimate partner violence in healthcare settings. Cochrane Database Syst Rev (7):CD007007

Patterson K, Grenny J, McMillan R, Switzler A (2012) Crucial conversations: tools for talking when stakes are high, 2nd edn. McGraw Hill, London

Radford L, Corral S, Bradley C, Fisher H, Bassett C, Howat N, Collishaw S (2011) Child abuse and neglect in the UK today. Research report. NSPCC, London

Ringrose J, Gill R, Livingstone S, Harvey L (2012) A qualitative study of children, young people and 'sexting': a report prepared for the NSPCC. NSPCC, London. http://eprints.lse. ac.uk/44216/1/__Libfile_repository_Content_Livingstone,%20S_A%20qualitative%20 study%20of%20children,%20young%20people%20and%20'sexting'%20(LSE%20RO).pdf. Accessed 20 June 2019

Sheridan L, Roberts K (2011) Key questions to consider in stalking cases. Behav Sci Law 29:255–270. https://doi.org/10.1002/bsl.966

Smith PH, White JW, Holland LJ (2003) A longitudinal perspective on dating violence among adolescent and college-age women. Am J Public Health 93(7):1104–1109

Smith E, Belton E, Barnard M, Fisher HL, Taylor J (2015) Strengthening the mother-child relationship following domestic abuse: service evaluation. Child Abuse Rev 24:261–273

Spangaro J, Poulos R, Zwi A (2011) Pandora doesn't live here anymore: normalization of screening for intimate partner violence in Australian antenatal, mental health and substance abuse services. Violence Vict 26:130–144

Sprague S, Madden K, Simunovic N, Godin K, Pham NK, Bhandari M (2012) Barriers to screening for intimate partner violence. Women Health 52(6):587–605

Stanley N (2011) Children experiencing domestic violence: a research review. Research in Practice, Dartington

Stanley N, Humphreys C (2017) Identifying the key components of a 'whole family' intervention for families experiencing domestic violence and abuse. J Gender Based Violence 1:99–115. https://doi.org/10.1332/239868017X14913081639164

Stonard KE, Bowen E, Lawrence TR, Shelley AP (2014) The relevance of technology to the nature, prevalence and impact of adolescent dating violence and abuse: a research synthesis. Aggress Violent Behav 19:390–417

Tarzia L, Humphreys C, Hegarty K (2017) Translating research about domestic and family violence into practice in Australia: possibilities and prospects. Evidence Policy 13(4):709–722

Thiara RK, Humphreys C (2017) Absent presence: the on-going impact of men's violence on the mother-child relationship. Child Family Social Work 22:137–145. https://doi.org/10.1111/cfs.12210

UNICEF and The Body Shop International (2006) Behind closed doors: the impact of domestic violence on children. London: UNICEF and The Body Shop International Plc. http://www.unicef.org/protection/files/BehindClosedDoors.pdf. Accessed 20 June 2019

Walby S, Towers J, Francis B (2014) Mainstreaming domestic and gender-based violence into sociology and the criminology of violence. Sociol Rev 62:187–214

Whitfield CL, Anda RF, Dube SR, Felitti VJ (2003) Violent childhood experiences and the risk of intimate partner violence in adults: assessment in a large health maintenance organization. J Interpers Violence 18(2):166–185

Older People and Domestic Violence and Abuse

Sarah Wydall and Elize Freeman

For sometime, global demographic trends have indicated that the continued growth of the ageing population is 'pervasive', 'unprecedented' and 'enduring' (United Nations 2002, 2018). In the UK, for example, it is estimated that by 2040 nearly one in four people will be aged 65 or over and the number of people aged 85 or over is predicted to more than double to over 3.2 million (Office for National Statistics 2017). The picture is similar in the US with forecasts that by 2035, there will be more older people than children (US Census Bureau 2018). In Japan, this is already the case and it has the world's most aged population with 33% aged 60 years or over (United Nations 2015). These unremitting global trends are having considerable economic, political, cultural and social implications (United Nations 2018). Despite women making up most of the older population in virtually all the world's populations, the needs of older women who experience DVA has received little attention (Zink et al. 2004). This chapter provides guidance for health professionals on how to respond effectively to domestic violence and abuse (DVA) in cases involving people aged 60 years and over. This chapter explores the impact DVA on the health and well-being of older people. The literature will highlight examples of how older victim-survivors of DVA are treated differently because of ageist and sexist socio-cultural misconceptions and stereotyping.

A key point to reflect on as a current or future health professional is to ensure you do not discriminate because of an individual's age, gender, sexuality, ethnicity, disability and support needs in cases of DVA. Both formal and informal working practices and cultures within your organisation can also influence how you treat people (Flynn and Citarella 2013). Constant professional development, training, evaluation and reflection about your practice will help safeguard against discrimination and

S. Wydall (✉) · E. Freeman
Dewis Choice, Centre for Age, Gender and Social Justice, Aberystwyth University,
Aberystwyth, UK
e-mail: sww@aber.ac.uk

© Springer Nature Switzerland AG 2020
P. Ali, J. McGarry (eds.), *Domestic Violence in Health Contexts: A Guide for Healthcare Professions*, https://doi.org/10.1007/978-3-030-29361-1_7

harm. In healthcare settings, it is particularly important that you do not patronise, infantilise or place less value in what an older person says to you when they disclose they are being mistreated and abused. For older victim-survivors who disclose DVA, **validation** of the abuse—i.e. being listened to, believed and taken seriously by a professional is crucial to improving their sense of well-being at a critical juncture in their lives (Wydall et al. 2019). The case studies, learning activities and reflective activities in this chapter will help you to ensure older people's rights; entitlements and experience of support are equal to those of their younger counterparts.

In the past, health professionals have often not recognised DVA as a health and well-being issue that occurs in later life (Van Hightower 2002); thus they may have only viewed as individuals through a biomedical lens and adopted a Cartesian reductivist approach for treatment. For health professionals today, it is important to adopt a holistic health model but also have an awareness of the health implications that may arise, both chronic and acute. For example, individuals are likely to experience chronic anxiety and depression as a consequence of the abuse and they may also present with numerous trauma—related injuries, gastrointestinal problems, joint pain, urinary and gynaecological issues. Furthermore, perpetrators often use sleep and food deprivation and/or withhold medication to control the victim-survivor. (Women's Aid 2007; McGarry et al. 2011; Wydall et al. 2019).

Later life is sometimes marked by increasing medicalisation and contact with a wide range of health professionals; consequently, there are many opportunities for health professionals to build a rapport with patients. Perpetrators will actively try to minimise the victim-survivors contact with people, thus missed appointments should be flagged up as a cause for concern. Professionals should be vigilant to a **performance of caring and attentive family** member(s) that may be masking a hyper-vigilant perpetrator(s) actively preventing the health professional speaking with a patient/client on their own. Even if the client states they want the perpetrator with them, they may have been threatened to insist that they want the relative with them when they want to seek help and disclose that they are at risk of harm. Thus, where you can, **always find a reason to speak with the client alone** in a safe and confidential environment.

If supported appropriately, many victim-survivors, irrespective of age, may choose to leave the abusive perpetrator, however this is their choice. Leaving is the most dangerous time in the relationship for victim-survivors and their family, as perpetrators are more likely to commit homicide if they sense the victim-survivor is separating from them either symbolically and/or physically (Dobash and Dobash 2015; Monckton-Smith et al. 2017). Furthermore, the abusive behaviours may escalate in the period **during and after** leaving the perpetrator, thus individuals need to be prepared and supported appropriately, as they move into a period of recovery and reestablish a sense of self, rebuilding social ties broken down by the abuser isolation tactics. Given the individual's complex range of needs at this point in their help-seeking journey, safety planning and a co-ordinated community response is crucial.

Good Practice Guidance
It is important that **you use the terms the person who discloses the abuse uses.** For example, if a women aged 84 years states she is arguing with her son and the women is upset because he hit her, use the same language as the victim-survivor uses and work to develop a relationship of trust that does not alienate you from engaging with her and her son. If you state this is 'domestic abuse' and her son is a perpetrator, not only will this lead to disengagement, it could prevent the individual from seeking help in the future. A proportionate response is crucial. Reflect that when an adult child is abusing a parent they are more likely to have tolerated the abuse for much longer and they are more likely to put the needs of their adult child before their own needs. Working within a multi-agency framework and seeking separate support for the adult child is more likely to result in a positive outcome than working in silo with your client/patient.

DVA impacts on individual's social, economic and environmental resources and these wider determinants of health influence the individual's mental and physical health needs (Marmot and Bell 2012; Postmus et al. 2018). If you are working as part of a co-ordinated community response you can help by good joint working with partners to increase a survivor's sense of *social capital as they recover (Gibson-Davis et al. 2005; Wydall et al. 2019). Moving to a new home and community setting, building self-esteem and gaining environmental mastery whilst trying to reconnect and restore relationships damaged by the abuser will influence the individual's sense of health and well-being, hence the need for a client-centred tailored package of support. Older people in particular will experience 'service poverty' when help-seeking in the context of domestic abuse, as such they often feel very alone, isolated and fearful. Thus helping to signpost victim-survivors to engage with a range of statutory and third sector services, will promote a sense of support and reduce feelings of isolation. Recovery is not a linear process and the impact of coercive control and experiencing multiple traumatic events will have severe psychological and physical impact on health. Health professionals have a key role in looking beyond clinical and biomedical factors to ensure they provide a holistic and empowering range of health provision to facilitate an enabling relationship. Health professionals will also be involved in safeguarding processes, so understanding domestic abuse risk assessment tools (Robbins et al. 2016) and contributing towards safety planning will help prevent further harms from perpetrators who will actively work against professional interventions in an attempt to maintain control. We will revisit perpetrator behaviours later on in the chapter when we discuss case studies. However, it is important to remind us that (a) coercive control is a feature in almost all cases of DVA. (b) Any family member can be a perpetrator, so whilst men are more likely to be perpetrators and women, their victims, anyone irrespective of gender, age, sexuality and class within a family group can perpetrate abuse targeting one or more family members. Thus, not only intimate partner's abuse, but sons, daughters or grandchildren, and in-laws as well as extended family can harm and abuse an older person. It is also important to note that more than one perpetrator can exist in a family network and that a perpetrator is unlikely to target just one victim-survivor. Thus across a family many people may be experiencing abuse∗ and coercive control, hence the need for good partnership communication and detailed note taking.

7.1   Key Facts About Domestic Abuse and Older People

Clients age in years	60 and under	Over 60
Perpetrator is current partner	28%	40%
Male clients	4%	21%
Adult family member is the primary perpetrator	6%	44%
Multiple perpetrators	9%	7%
Average length of abuse	4 years	6.5 years
Physical health & mental health	6 and 7	6 and 6
Physical abuse	69%	69%
Sexual abuse	25%	10%[a]
Harassment and stalking	73%	57%
Jealous and controlling behaviours	83%	73%

Adapted from SafeLives, U.K. 2016. Safe Later Lives:
Older People and Domestic Abuse, Spotlights Report
[a]Less likely to disclose sexual abuse

The chart above is drawn from one of the largest datasets in England and Wales that includes a sample of older people. However, the data only provide an indication of some of the similarities and differences in relation to age of the victim-survivor with individuals who have reported DVA. It is important to note that older people are less likely to disclose sexual abuse, but this does not mean they have not experienced it; they just may **require more time** to share this feature of the abusive relationship. Furthermore, interpreting the data inaccurately can create false assumptions about individual choices. For example, a lack of available services will inhibit help-seeking which will increase the time the older person endures the abuse and potentially increase the risk∗. Note that one in four domestic homicides occurs in people aged 60 years and over. There is now significant evidence to show that older people are as likely to experience DVA as their younger counterparts are, but less likely to report it. Why is this?

7.2   'Myths, Stereotypes and Ageism and a Lack of Service Provision'

In the UK, three generations of people aged over 60 years are often artificially separated into distinct groups for heuristic purposes. The grouping by generation provides only an indication of how life experiences may influence attitudes and beliefs. For professionals, this grouping helps to highlight that older people are not a homogenous group (all the same) but these generational differences are only a small part of the jigsaw that determines human behaviours and decision-making. People aged 60 years and over comprised of three generations of people and there is as much variation in attitudes and health needs both within and across generations as with other age groups.

> Born 1901–1927 (colloquially known as the GI generation [USA])
> Characteristics: The idea that marriage was for life
> Women were expected to take on caring roles rather than go out to work
> Respect and deference for (male) authority

> Born 1928–1945 (The silent generation)
> Characteristics: The experience of World War 2 led to a 'make do and mend' approach
> Sacrifice and a strong work ethos were valued
> Divorce was extremely rare and children born out of wedlock were stigmatised
> Increasing emphasis was placed on the differing roles of women and men

> Born 1946–1964 (The baby boomers)
> Growing up in the 1960s and 1970s a time of significant social, cultural and political change
> The pill gave women and men increasing choice and freedom
> First UK women's refuge (1971)
> Shift in attitudes towards marriage and divorce

When you think about your own generation, you may be aware that whilst you and your friends may share similar views on climate change or views on marriage, parenting or education you are also aware of the vast differences in behaviours and attitudes when you discuss certain topic areas or make choices about your life.

Born 1965–1994 Generation X&Y

Moved from an analog childhood and teenage years to see significant developments in an adult digital age

Experienced periods of growth and societal shifts in perception towards young people, a growing awareness of LGBTQ groups and BAME issues

However, with significant changes in the Labour Market, England and Wales experienced mass unemployment, and the rise of the YUPPIE and a renewed focus on individualism

Everyone's worldview is unique. This 'uniqueness' is in part influenced by your childhood, family background, socioeconomic status, culture, education and the peer groups and social networks you are exposed to throughout your life course. Thus, the three generations of people aged 60 and over will have had multiple life events and individual challenges, but each individual will have come through these experiences in a unique way and their viewpoints and the decisions they make will be distinctive.

Born 1995–2012

Generation Z. Could this be you?

Shuns conformity and tradition so marriage no longer viewed as key feature in life course

Individual development and experience is prioritised

Entrepreneurial and tech savvy, able to multitask but with shorter attention spans

For future health professionals, it is important that you treat everyone equally as individuals and provide the same opportunities and choices to people irrespective of their age. However, you need to be aware of the barriers in policy and practice that discriminate against certain people, so you can challenge these barriers and work to ensure people in your profession and in other professions respond appropriately. The next section will explore how ageism has impacted on policy and practice in the area of domestic abuse.

7.3   Domestic Violence and Abuse and the Public Story of Domestic Violence and Abuse

Certain demographic groups who experience DVA fall outside the 'picture' presented by the society as **who may be a victim-survivor of DVA**. So, if you think about DVA, the imagery and the language used to raise awareness and direct people to services reflects what is a narrow demographic, the 'public story of domestic abuse' i.e. the victim is white, female, heterosexual, under 40 years of age, with young children. Very few images depict men, people of colour, LGBTQ+, disability and younger or older people as victim-survivors. Similarly, perpetrators are portrayed as young, white, heterosexual males if they are visible at all. As images of older people are not often used in public health campaigns about domestic abuse, it is difficult for older men and women to see themselves as potential victims of domestic abuse. It is a sad reflection of our ageist society that most imagery of older people often only presents stereotyped photos of wrinkly hands, rather than older faces, mobility aids and people seated with a health professional or similar standing above them and touching them with a reassuring pat. The lack of demographic diversity in the imagery used and the invisibility of older faces serves to instil in society a false perception of ageing as a period of physiological decline, a loss of engagement with social networks and isolation. This negative framing of later life is known as the 'decline' analogy characterised by disengagement and physiological decline (Cummings and Henry 1961) and this is the dominant social construction of ageing in Western society. This negative construction of older people has consequences for the majority of individuals aged 60 years and over who want help and support to stop the abuse. Many of the stereotypical assumptions about older people's life choices and behaviours may serve to mask the signs of domestic abuse. Thus, in the domestic homicide reviews of older people, it is evident that health professionals have applied a 'rule of optimism' about later life and caring roles and failed to ask, act and safeguard the individual experiencing domestic abuse (Sharp-Jeffs and Kelly 2016; Wydall et al. 2018).

Furthermore, because later in life is often highly medicalised and the relationship between patient and professional can be hierarchical rather than collaborative (Illich 1975; Anderson 1995) health professionals may inadvertently treat an older person as a passive recipient of care. Professionals may assume people are incapable of making an informed choice and act on their behalf. Such infantilisation further impacts on the individual's ability to seek help, ask for support and trust in professional's responses. Invalidating an individual's disclosure of harm could lead to serious implications as in the case of Mr. C (please see Box 7.1).

Box 7.1
Summary: Unlawful killing of Mr. C by his partner. The panel concluded that Mr. C had been assaulted at least over a period of months and probably years. He was physically, emotionally and financially abused. The panel identified a key practice episode when Mr. C did disclose, but health professionals **did not respond proactively**, only addressing his immediate health needs but not prioritising his safety nor attending to his health and well-being.

Issues identified: Mr. C's family knew of some of the abuse but were unable to convince Mr. C to seek help or leave Mr. Y. It may be that being an older gay man may have made it more difficult for Mr. C to seek help and for professionals to identify the assault as domestic abuse. Mr. C's problematic alcohol use appears to have been allowed to mask the signs of abuse, even when he disclosed. **The many health professionals that Mr. C saw in the last year of his life did not pick up the signs of abuse or ask about it.** http://www.safeinthecity.info/published-domestic-homicide-reviews 2014

Time to Reflect
Thinking about older people and nursing practice, how do you think older people are seen by healthcare professionals these days? What can you do in your future practice to change discriminatory practice?

7.4 Systemic Invisibility: Older People, Ignored and Overlooked by Researchers, Policy Makers and Practitioners

The issue of DVA in later life has been largely ignored and overlooked by policy makers and researchers and this has influenced the rate of change in the development of services (SafeLives, U.K. 2016). Whilst there have been significant advances in our understanding in the last three decades about the causes and the consequences of DVA, the research and learning about has been drawn from age groups mainly below 60 years. Paternalistic attitudes about notions of 'vulnerability' also serve to act as a barrier to people engaging in research. For example, ethical guidance places further restrictions on capturing the views of certain groups of people. Gatekeepers also inhibit researcher's access to older people, thus denying them the choice to share their perceptions, not only of individual level barriers, but the importance of barriers within and across organisations both within the statutory, third sector and in wider society (Davies et al. 2009; Wydall et al. 2019).

Many research designs and subsequent fieldwork research tools have discriminated against older people when aiming to capture the prevalence of DVA. For example, the Crime Survey for England and Wales (CSEW) did not include DVA statistics for people over the age of 59 until April 2017. Whilst the age limit for those who can participate in the survey responses was raised to 74 years of age, this still excludes people over 75 years from one of the largest self-report victimisation study in Europe. Whilst there are exceptions, (McGarry et al. 2011; SafeLives, U.K. 2016; Dewis Choice 2015), very few research studies, both qualitative and/or quantitative, have included older people in their sample when examining the lived experiences of people experiencing DVA. Therefore, the lack of empirical research has limited our understanding of DVA across three generations of people aged 60 years and over. This paucity of evidence has also resulted in gaps in knowledge about the health and well-being implications of long-term or late onset abuse. As a result, policy makers tend to lack the necessary information to develop policies and plan strategically to target service development, which in turn influences the allocation of resources, thus narrowing the lens that defines who is a victim-survivor of domestic abuse and inhibiting the development of effective responses. When examining policy guidance, very little attention is given to groups who fall outside 'the public story', so in the case of older people, such systemic invisibility impacts on resources thus inhibiting older people's ability to seek help and make informed choices.

7.5   Do Older People Seek Help?

Research to date highlights that people aged 60 years and over who are victim-survivors of DVA experience discriminatory responses when they attempt to seek help from formal agencies when compared to people aged 59 years and under (Williams et al. 2013; Wydall and Zerk 2015). So why does age influence the quality of support received so significantly? The following factors influence service responses:

7.5.1   Services Diverting Older People Away from a Domestic Abuse Response

If you **are under 60** you are seen as a victim of DVA, therefore you are usually directed down a criminal justice response but also provided with access to welfare support. Therefore, you have access to resources to help with housing, mental health, benefits, and civil and criminal justice responses. You will be risk assessed using a domestic abuse risk assessment tool and safety planning should take place to help keep you safe. However, if you are **60 years and over,** evidence suggests practitioners will not recognise DVA and coercive control in later life, thus they will divert the older person towards a **'welfarised'** response (Clarke et al. 2016). 'Welfarisation' denies people aged 60 years and over the choice to engage with DVA resources, and this is age discrimination. This means older people will be less likely to be risk assessed using domestic abuse risk assessment tools, and more likely to experience a single agency response (silo-working) which will be insufficient to meet the complex needs of a victim-survivor. A welfarised response will not only increase the risk of ongoing abuse and increase the likelihood of harm, but will also deny the individual access to domestic abuse resources and limit their choices.

Access to justice and appropriate domestic abuse risk assessments will help the individual gain access to resources that are tailored to provide a more holistic service. As part of a co-ordinated community response, health professionals need to be aware how to access a range of agencies that are trained to manage risk and safety issues associated with DVA. The welfarisation of older victim-survivors may be one of the reasons why many older people stay with the abuser because they do not have the necessary support in place to help them make an informed choice nor are they made aware of the possible civil and criminal options available to hold perpetrators accountable. The table below provides some insights into older people's experiences and the multiple barriers they may face when seeking help (See also Wydall and Zerk 2017).

What we know so far about people aged 60 and over experiencing DVA
Like their younger counterparts, older people:

- Will be aware that a formal disclosure significantly increases the risk of homicide and increased harm to themselves and other family members
- May not recognise the abuse as domestic abuse nor will they understand coercive control as a perpetrator tactic;

- May wish to leave or stay with the perpetrator and it is important they are supported through their help-seeking journey;
- May experience discrimination from services and victim-blaming attitudes from professionals who do not understand domestic abuse;
- Minimise the range of abuses they experience and make excuses for the perpetrator's behaviours;
- May need time and space to learn how to decide for themselves as they may be unused to making decisions or they may have learnt to doubt their own judgement.

7.5.2 There Is a Poverty of Service Provision Aimed at Supporting Male and Female Victims-Survivors

As services do not advertise that they support older people, especially men, people who are LGBTQ+ and those from BME background are unlikely to enter these premises and seek help. However, older people may not want to use terms such as domestic abuse to describe the abuse they are experiencing, especially if it is from an adult child, thus the use of appropriate language and imagery is key to stimulating the uptake of services for three generations of people aged 60 years and over.

7.6 Good Practice Example

There are a growing number of services that provide dedicated support to people aged 60, and over experiencing domestic abuse in the United Kingdom. The next section will provide an insight into one of these services and provide some case study examples.

7.6.1 Dewis Choice

Dewis Choice, a service in Dyfed Powys, Wales is comprised of both a service and a research strand. The initial model for the service was developed through community-based participatory action research. However, as so little was known about the needs of older men and women in the context of domestic abuse, the model is a work in progress informed by qualitative data from the longitudinal research element of the project. The service Dewis Choice provides is client-centred, working with individuals, families and where it is safe to do so, harmers to support people aged 60 and over. The principal ethos of the approach is to be client-led, to integrate justice, well-being, prevention, and recovery work and promote empowerment through listening to older victim-survivors.

The service element of Dewis Choice consists of two Choice Support workers and a Well-being practitioner. Co-located within third sector specialist domestic abuse settings, referrals to Dewis Choice come via social services. Working within such infrastructures reduces the likelihood of clients left without support and improves information sharing and inter-agency communication.

The two Choice Support workers are trained IDSVAs (Independent Domestic, Sexual Violence Advisor-Safe Lives), like IDSVAs their purpose is to address the safety of the victim-survivors working within a multi-agency framework. However, the role is distinct from an IDSVA, as workers not only address immediate safety needs, they may work together in parallel with harmers, clients and other family members adopting a whole family approach. In addition, the service involves intensive support for up to a 12-month period for clients who deemed to be a standard risk, according to the Domestic Abuse, Stalking and Harassment and Honour-Based Violence Risk Identification Checklist (DASH-RIC) (Safe Lives 2014).

The Choice Support workers not only explore civil, criminal and restorative options, they also introduce the client to a Well-being practitioner. The Well-being practitioner identifies how harmers have negatively influenced either directly or indirectly, a client's well-being and provides strategies to help them and their families overcome the impact of DVA. The well-being element of the service was developed from the Community-based PAR, focus groups and analysis of client's and practitioner's qualitative data. The Well-being practitioner uses a co-ordinated community response to engage with a range of other agencies, including health, housing, the police and community groups.

The Dewis Choice service provides support for all people aged 60 years and over including those who lack mental capacity. It does not, at this stage in the pilot offer support to those in institutional settings such as care/nursing homes or hospices.

The prospective longitudinal study aims to capture the lived experiences of older people during their help-seeking journey. To date the empirical findings, provide some insights into the experience of domestic abuse in later life. The priorities listed below will help to promote service engagement and the case studies will identify key areas of well-being for health and social care professionals to be aware of:

Priorities
- The voice of the older person is paramount—listen to them and act accordingly
- Older people must be able to speak freely without coercion
- Information must be provided in an appropriate form to enable the older person to make an informed decision
- Older people must be made aware of their human rights and all their entitlements

Help-seeking, a continuous and nonlinear journey—Health professionals should:

- Recognise the courage required to begin to seek help
- Work with the client to tackle stress, anxiety and low feelings of self-esteem
- Show empathy and support in all instances

- Families can provide strong support, however, intensive advocacy work is necessary to explore the family dynamics and the nature of the abuse
- Be aware of the importance of identifying coercive and controlling behaviour
- The client/patients' priorities will shift over time as part of the recovery process
- Clients/patients may leave the abuser more than once before finally leaving, do not judge them and support them more as they work through these significant life challenges
- Needs, wishes and the support required frequently fall outside existing set models

7.7 Case Studies and Links to Guidance on Domestic Abuse

7.7.1 Responding to a Long-Term Intimate Partner Domestic Abuse: Lillian, 83

Lillian aged 83 years old, was referred to Dewis Choice by a Domestic Abuse Officer from the police. Lillian initially came to the attention of health services on admittance to hospital following a fall in her home. Lillian had osteoarthritis in her spine; impairing her mobility. Blood cell counts confirmed she was anaemic.

Lillian later described how her husband of 62 years, John, a retired GP aged 85, refused her requests to call neighbours or paramedics when she fell. John administered sedatives, which had not been prescribed for Lillian, as she lay on the floor, in excess of 8 h. When John finally called for assistance, Lillian described seeing the "shock" on the Paramedics faces as they observed living conditions in the property due to John's hoarding behaviour.

What staff did
- **Hospital staff raised concerns about John's behaviour towards Lillian**, noting, when John was present, Lillian would appear agitated "changing her mind to agree with whatever he said." John was verbally abusive towards staff, demanding they discharge Lillian into his care.
- Paramedics and hospital staff identified **Lillian as being an "Adult at risk"** (Legislation.gov.uk 2014), and **proactively followed safeguarding procedures, making separate referrals to Local Authority Adult Safeguarding.**

What staff did not do
- Hospital staff were **not proactive in identifying Lillian as a victim-survivor of domestic abuse.**
- Hospital staff neglected **to actively engage in discussion with Lillian** about John's behaviour, **a missed opportunity for her to disclose further information** (Safelives.org.uk 2016).
- Lillian **was not offered the support of a specialist domestic abuse** practitioner at this stage.

The next steps
- Adult Social Services carried out **a care assessment** and decided not to discharge Lillian to her home, **proposing a temporary admittance to residential care for recovery respite**.

Discriminatory practice
- The response of Health, Adult Safeguarding and Adult Social Care was to initiate only a welfarised approach to Lillian, thus prioritising immediate health, care and welfare needs. They did not at this stage, **provide access to DVA resources**, such as a hospital based or external IDVA (Independent Domestic Violence Advisor), with knowledge of domestic abuse procedures, who could undertake a DASH (Domestic Abuse Stalking Homicide) assessment to measure the risks. By not working with Lillian, Lillian was put in the position of a 'passive observer,' with minimal control or input to decision-making processes. **Ageist assumptions** and a **lack of understanding** of older people experiencing domestic abuse can result in practitioners instigating a welfarised approach in isolation, denying older people access to the domestic abuse support offered to a younger person (Clarke et al. 2016).

7.7.2   What Happened Next?

Hospital staff contacted Lillian's son and daughter-in-law, who agreed to take Lillian and John to live in their home, providing respite support for Lillian. Lillian's son explained later to the Dewis choice Practitioner that, although he had been aware his father was a 'manipulative and controlling individual', he did not have sufficient understanding of domestic abuse to recognise his father's behaviour as coercive control or realise the risks he posed to Lillian and his family until later. At the point of referral to Dewis Choice, John had returned to his home without Lillian. Lillian's son had contacted police when John returned, attempting to break into their property to retrieve Lillian, despite her now stating clearly she wanted no further contact with him. John has since made two attempts to use safeguarding referrals to gain access to Lillian, claiming she has dementia and lacks capacity, resulting in Lillian having to undergo a mental capacity assessment.

What went wrong next?
- The police referral **did not indicate physical abuse**, despite the administration of medication by John, as this information **had not been shared** between Police and Safeguarding Teams when Lillian moved to a new local authority.

Next steps
- The Dewis Choice Well-being Practitioner, a qualified IDVSA (Independent domestic and sexual violence advisor), met with Lillian and identified Lillian was fearful of statutory services as she believed they had the power to send her back to John. Lillian's son was also fearful he would be accused of influencing Lillian. The family described how they felt 'under siege'.

7.7.3 Client-Centred Approach

The Dewis Choice Practitioner worked with Lillian and the family to increase their understanding of the roles and remit of statutory services and Lillian's right to control over her decision-making about where she lived, who she had contact with and her ongoing care and support.

What took place?
- The Dewis Choice Practitioner **helped the family form a safety plan,** including measures that Lillian was not left in the home alone, external doors were to be kept locked, the grandchildren understood not to open the door to John, and the address was flagged with local police for a quick response.
- The Dewis Choice Practitioner **discussed abusive behaviours with Lillian and the family.** Lillian and her son recognised they had both experienced coercive control by John, and her daughter-in-law felt more confident to offer support and discuss abuse with Lillian.
- Lillian told the Dewis Choice Practitioner she looked forward to her visiting as she felt understood by her and trusted her expert knowledge of domestic abuse. Over time **Lillian disclosed that John had always been controlling** and, as her mobility declined, she became more fearful of John and aware of the risks he posed to her physical safety, which led to her experiencing increased anxiety and panic attacks. Whilst in hospital John had told Lillian, if she fell again, he would not call paramedics as there had been 'consequences'. Lillian had been terrified of being discharged home with John but had not felt able to voice her fears and no one had asked.
- The Dewis Choice Practitioner discussed with Lillian the **criminal option** of obtaining a restraining order and **civil option** of obtaining a non-molestation order, should John persist in attempting to access her. Lillian did not want to pursue a complaint of assault against John but following a **discussion of her rights**, asked for support to pursue a divorce and financial settlement.

Over a 6-month period, Lillian became more self-assured, angry and assertive, demonstrating increased confidence in her ability and right to make her own decisions. Lillian's mobility improved with support from occupational therapy and physiotherapy. Her physical health improved with blood tests showing her cell count returning to normal.

7.8   Case Study Two

7.8.1   Multi-Agency Response to Adult Familial Abuse: Deborah, 75

Deborah, aged 75, was referred to Dewis Choice by a Community Practice Nurse when she disclosed experiencing financial abuse by her eldest son. The Nurse explained, Deborah had been attending the community hospital for support with mobility and diabetes since moving to the area to live with the eldest of her three sons 2 years previously. Prior to this Deborah had lived with her youngest son and his wife.

What staff did

- The Practice Nurse **recognised that Deborah was experiencing domestic abuse** from her son and contacted Dewis choice for advice.
- The Practice Nurse **explained** to Deborah how Dewis Choice could support her and **asked for Deborah's permission** to refer her to Dewis Choice.
- The Practice Nurse **arranged for Deborah to meet the Dewis Choice Practitioner at the community hospital**, so her son was not aware Deborah was meeting with a domestic abuse advisor.

7.8.2   What Happened Next?

Deborah met the Dewis Choice Practitioner and disclosed she had also experienced abuse from her youngest son and daughter-in-law during the 10 years she had lived in the annex she had paid to have built on their home. Deborah's son and daughter-in-law had taken complete control of Deborah's finances, denying her access to her pension and care allowance. Deborah's daughter-in-law had been emotionally abusive and controlled Deborah's daily movements including when she could go to bed and get up, and what she could eat. Deborah had no privacy or control over her personal space. When Deborah confided in her eldest son, he persuaded her to move in with him. However, he immediately took control of Deborah's bank account, and claimed carer's allowance for Deborah despite providing no care.

7.8.3   Client-Centred Approach

The Dewis Choice Practitioner explored Deborah's options with her and she identified she wanted to live independently, but remain in the local area as she had supportive networks within the local community.

Multi-agency working—best practice

- The Practitioner worked with the Practice Nurse to form **a multi-agency response** with Health, Occupational Therapy, Housing, Social Services and Benefits advisors. They were able **to support Deborah's** application for housing, ensuring she was recognised as having homeless status as she was fleeing domestic abuse.
- Deborah was **allocated sheltered housing** and an occupational therapy assessment was arranged to ensure it was suitable.
- The Dewis Choice Practitioner formed an **individualised safety plan** with Deborah, taking account of her mobility and health needs, ensuring Deborah always had enough money for a taxi, a mobile phone charged with emergency contact numbers, and a small supply of her medication on her person. With Deborah's permission **the plan was shared with health practitioners,** with whom she was in regular contact, and Deborah's middle son, whom Deborah identified as safe.

The next steps

- Deborah's move was carefully managed and once she was settled in her new home, she felt **ready to explore justice options.** Deborah asked for help to go through her financial records to assess the extent of the financial abuse before deciding whether to report to police. Deborah asked for help arranging a solicitor's appointment to see if she could recover the money she had spent on the annex to her youngest son's home.

Reflecting on the process the Practice nurse explained she initially had reservations around Deborah living independently and was surprised by the subsequent improvement in her mobility. Deborah became actively engaged in several community groups and demonstrated increased confidence in managing her home and finances. The diabetic nurse reported that Deborah was managing her diabetes more consistently than over the past 2 years.

7.8.4   Summary

This chapter introduced domestic abuse as a concept and provided an insight into the significant impact of domestic abuse on the health and well-being of older people. The literature has highlighted examples of how older victim-survivors of DVA experience discrimination. As a current or future health professional, the chapter has drawn attention to where discrimination had led to a safeguarding issue because an individual's age, gender, sexuality, ethnicity, disability and support needs has led to an inappropriate response. Be aware that formal and informal working practices and cultures within your organisation can also influence how you treat people and so always report abuse. Constant professional development, training in the area of domestic abuse, coercive control, risk assessment and safety planning, self-evaluation and reflection about your practice will help safeguard against discrimination and harm and ensure you provide the most effective response in cases of domestic abuse in later life.

Summary Points

- **Create a safe space** for one to one discussion; reassure the older person that you will not share information with their family members unless they ask you to do so.
- **Validation and Positive Action**—always listen to the client, take their concerns seriously and act. Remember Mr. C and the Domestic Homicide Review which suggested Mr. C disclosed on several occasions, but health professionals placed more value in what his carer (the perpetrator) said about his injuries and his behaviour than they placed in Mr. C's disclosure of the abuse.
- **Disclosure and asking the questions**—always use the terms the older person uses to define the abuse they are experiencing and ask about the relationship and the wider family network to establish a fuller picture of the client's circumstances. Move at the pace of the individual, avoid interrupting the clients reflect back on what you have heard and clarify to ensure you have heard correctly what

has been said. Take time to develop a rapport to explore what the client does and doesn't want, remembering that their priorities may change over time.

- **Ask yourself, are you or other agencies making ageist assumptions about the individual's choices?** Are you giving the older person the correct advice? Ensure that older people are offered parity of services similar to the options offered to a younger person, and ensure that older people are in a position to make an informed choice.
- **Do not make assumptions about someone's capacity and ability to engage** based on age-related health conditions. For example, an undiagnosed hearing impairment may lead to inaccurate assumptions about an individual's level of understanding.
- **Always avoid the 'rule of optimism'**—do not assume family members are acting in the best interests of the older relative (see Wydall et al. 2018).

Web Resources

Legislation.gov.uk (2014) Care act 2014 [online]. http://www.legislation.gov.uk/ukpga/2014/23/pdfs/ukpga_20140023_en.pdf. Accessed 3 April 2019

https://www.scie.org.uk/

Safelives.org.uk (2016) A Cry for Health Why we must invest in domestic abuse services in hospitals [online]. http://www.safelives.org.uk/sites/default/files/resources/SAFJ4993_Themis_report_WEBcorrect.pdf. Accessed 3 April 2019

Unlocking stories: older women's experiences of domestic violence and abuse told through creative expression. http://www.nottingham.ac.uk/helmopen/rlos/safeguarding/unlocking-stories/

Bibliography

Abrahams H (2007) Supporting women after domestic violence: loss, trauma and recovery. Jessica Kingsley Publishing, London

Davies M, Rogers P (2009) Perceptions of blame and credibility toward victims of childhood sexual abuse: differences across victim age, victim-perpetrator relationship, and respondent gender in a depicted case. J Child Sexual Abuse 18(1):78–92

Donovan C, Hester M (2014) Domestic violence and sexuality: what's love got to do with it? Policy Press, Bristol

Groves N, Thomas T (2013) Domestic violence and the criminal justice system. Routledge, Oxon

Home Office (2011) Crime in England and Wales 2010/11: findings from the British crime survey and police recorded crime. https://assets.publishing.service.gov.uk/government/uploads/system/uploads/attachment_data/file/116417/hosb1011.pdf

Home Office (2013) Domestic violence and abuse: new definition. http://www.homeoffice.gov.uk/crime/violence-against-women-girls/domestic-violence/

Home Office (2016) Domestic violence and abuse. Guidance: domestic violence and abuse. https://www.gov.uk/guidance/domestic-violence-and-abuse

Kelly L (1988) Surviving sexual violence (feminist perspectives). Polity Press, Oxford

Kelly L (2003) The wrong debate: reflections on why force is not the key issue with respect to trafficking in women for sexual exploitation. Fem Rev 73:139–144

Kelly L, Sharp N, Klein R (2014) Finding the costs of freedom: how women and children rebuild their lives after domestic violence. Solace Women's Aid, London

McGarry J, Simpson C (2011) Domestic abuse and older women: exploring the opportunities for service development and care delivery. J Adult Prot 13(6):294–301

Myhill A (2015) Measuring coercive control: what can we learn from national population surveys? Violence Against Women 21(3):355–375

Pence E, McMahon M (1997) A coordinated community response to domestic violence. Unpublished manuscript, Duluth Domestic Abuse Intervention Project, Duluth

Postmus JL, Hoge G, Breckenridge J, Sharp-Jeffs N, Chung D (2018) Economic abuse as an invisible form of domestic violence: a multicounty review. Trauma Violence Abuse. Advanced online publication. https://doi.org/10.1177/1524838018764160

SafeLives UK (2014) SafeLives Dash risk checklist for the identification of high risk cases of domestic abuse, stalking and 'honour'-based violence. http://www.safelives.org.uk/sites/default/files/resources/YP%20RIC%20guidance%20FINAL%20%281%29.pdf.   Accessed 07.09.2019

Stark E (2007) Coercive control: how men entrap women in personal life. Oxford University Press, New York

The Office of National Statistics (2017). https://www.ons.gov.uk/peoplepopulationandcommunity/crimeandjustice/bulletins/domesticabuseinenglandandwales/yearendingmarch2017

Van Hightower NR, Gorton J (2002) A case study of community-based responses to rural woman battering. Violence Against Women 8(7):845–872

Williams J, Wydall S, Clarke A (2013) Protecting older victims of abuse who lack capacity: the role of the independent mental capacity advocate. Elder Law Review 2(3):167–174

Women's Aid (2007) Older women and domestic violence: an overview

Wydall S, Clarke A, Williams J, Zerk R (2019) Dewis choice: a Welsh Initiative promoting justice for older victim-survivors of domestic abuse. In: Bows H (ed) Violence against older women: responses, 24 Palgrave Studies in Victims and Victimology, vol 2, 1st edn. Springer Nature, New York, pp 13–36

Bibliography

Anderson RM (1995) Patient empowerment and the traditional medical model: a case of irreconcilable differences? Diabetes Care 18(3):412–415

Clarke A, Williams J, Wydall S (2016) Access to justice for victims/survivors of elder abuse: a qualitative study. Soc Policy Soc 15(2):207–220

Cummings E, Henry WE (1961) Growing old and the process of disengagement. New York, Basic Book

Dobash R, Dobash R (2015) When men murder women (interpersonal violence). Oxford, New York

Flynn M, Citarella V (2013) Winterbourne view hospital: a glimpse of the legacy. J Adult Prot 15(4):173–181

Gibson-Davis CM, Magnuson K, Gennetian LA, Duncan GJ (2005) Employment and the risk of domestic abuse among low-income women. J Marriage Fam 67(5):1149–1168

Illich I (1975) The medicalization of life. J Med Ethics 1(2):73–77

Marmot M, Bell R (2012) Fair society, healthy lives. Public Health 126:S4–S10

McGarry J, Simpson C, Hinchliff-Smith K (2011) The impact of domestic abuse for older women: a review of the literature. Health Soc Care Community 19(1):3–14

Monckton-Smith J, Szymanska K, Haile S (2017) Exploring the relationship between stalking and homicide. Suzy Lamplugh Trust, London

Postmus J. L, Hoge G, Breckenridge J, Sharp-Jeffs N, & Chung D, (2018). Economic abuse as an invisible form of domestic violence: A multicounty review. Trauma, Violence, & Abuse. Advanced online publication. https://doi.org/10.1177/1524838018764160

Robbins R, Banks C, McLaughlin H, Bellamy C, Thackray D (2016) Is domestic abuse an adult social work issue? Soc Work Educ 35(2):131–143

SafeLives, U.K. (2016) Safe later Lives: older people and domestic abuse, spotlights report

Sharp-Jeffs N, Kelly L (2016) Domestic homicide review (DHR) case analysis: report for standing together report for standing together against domestic violence, available online at: Van Hightower, N.R. and Gorton, J., 2002. A case study of community-based responses to rural woman battering. Violence Against Women 8(7):845–872

United Nations (2002) World population ageing: 1950–2050. United Nations, New York

United Nations (2015) World population ageing. http://www.un.org/en/development/desa/population/publications/pdf/ageing/WPA2015_Report.pdf

United Nations (2018) Ageing. http://www.un.org/en/sections/issues-depth/ageing/

US Census Bureau (2018) Older people projected to outnumber children for first time in U.S. history. Release number CB18–41. https://www.census.gov/newsroom/press-releases/2018/cb18-41-population-projections.html

Wydall S, Zerk R (2015) Crimes against, and abuse of, older people in wales–access to support and justice: working together. Office of Older People's Commissioner for Wales, Cardiff. www.olderpeoplewales.com/en/adult_protection/aberystwyth_report.aspx

Wydall S, Zerk R (2017) Domestic abuse and older people: factors influencing help-seeking. J Adult Prot 19(5):247–260

Wydall S, Clarke A, Williams J, Zerk R (2018) Domestic abuse and elder abuse in Wales: a tale of two initiatives. Br J Soc Work 48(4):962–981

Zink T, Jacobson C, Regan S, Fisher B, Pabst S (2004) Hidden victims: the healthcare needs and experiences of older women in abusive relationships. J Women's Health 13(8):898–908

Domestic Violence and Abuse and Hidden Groups

8

Michaela Rogers

8.1 Introduction

Societies around the world are characterised by diversity and this diversity reflects a wide range of social characteristics, backgrounds and experiences. Despite this widespread diversity, many communities face marginalisation, social exclusion and, subsequently, they can be considered hidden or hard-to-reach (Ahmed and Rogers 2016). These are those communities who are often absent from mainstream discourse, research, policy and practice because of processes of invisibilisation or systemic exclusion that result from practices or structures that uphold systemic exclusion (Wilkerson et al. 2014). In this chapter, attention is given to some of these hard-to-reach communities, who can be invisible in policy, practice and research concerning domestic violence and abuse (DVA). This chapter will enable the reader to see beyond the 'public story' of DVA as it is well established that DVA is a complex global phenomenon affecting a concerningly high number of individuals and families, occurring across cultural, ethnic, religious, age and gender boundaries (WHO 2017). This chapter will explore current understandings about DVA in relation to the following groups of people who can be considered to be hard-to-reach within the context of DVA. This includes: lesbian, gay, bisexual, trans and queer (LGBTQ) communities; male victims; women with learning disabilities; black and ethnic minority (BME) communities.

The term hard-to-reach is a contested and ambiguous one (Cook 2002), however, it is frequently used within the fields of health and social care and in relation to health and social inequalities. In this way, hard-to-reach refers to those groups in society who experience distinct barriers to inclusion, participation and access to services (Flanagan and Hancock 2010). In the UK, for example, it is widely recognised that

M. Rogers (✉)
Department of Sociological Studies, University of Sheffield, Sheffield, UK
e-mail: m.rogers@sheffield.ac.uk

© Springer Nature Switzerland AG 2020
P. Ali, J. McGarry (eds.), *Domestic Violence in Health Contexts: A Guide for Healthcare Professions*, https://doi.org/10.1007/978-3-030-29361-1_8

cultural and social conditions have resulted in various groups being considered as hard-to-reach, including people who are asylum seekers or refugees, people from black and ethnic minority communities, and people from gender and sexual minority communities. Within the discourse of DVA, there is a dominant 'public story' that promotes the idea that there is a particular type of 'victim-survivor' and a particular type of 'perpetrator'. This public story perpetuates the myth that DVA is a problem of heterosexual male violence against heterosexual females of childbearing age (Donovan and Hester 2014). This has resulted in the exclusion of groups of people who do not easily fit into this typology. There are additional processes in operation which mean that some groups are marginalised, and therefore hidden or hard-to-reach, in the context of DVA. For example, an analysis of DVA as a problem for white populations highlights structural issues, such as gender inequality (Stark 2007), but when turning the lens to BME populations, DVA can be explained as resulting from cultural differences. This is problematic as it can result in othering processes, and the neglect of a focus on DVA within these communities.

8.2   Background: Policy and Practice

Before moving to discuss each hard-to-reach group, it is useful to consider how the policy framework for DVA addresses the issues faced by people who are victim-survivors of DVA and categorised as being from hard-to-reach populations. Policy responses in the UK should be underpinned by a Central Government initiative, the *Ending Violence against Women and Girls Strategy 2016–2020* (EVAWG) (Home Office 2016). This strategy states that all fields of practice should commit to tackling DVA as this is 'everyone's responsibility' (Home Office 2016: 11). The EVAWG strategy has three key target areas which are prevention, early help and increased reporting. Recognising the additional demands that this places on services in addition to the need to target hard-to-reach populations, the EVAWG documents reports that additional funding will be provided to support 'women from BME backgrounds, and innovative services for the most vulnerable with complex needs' (Home Office 2016: 11). There is, however, no mandate on commissioners or decision-makers on a localised basis to prioritise income for DVA services and resource-based challenges (such as competition for funding, piecemeal and short-term funding arrangements) persist (Rogers 2016). This is especially the case for agencies seeking to support hard-to-reach populations. For example, services for BME women, despite being described as 'lifelines', are often patchy and lack sustainability (Manjoo 2015).

The EVAWG strategy states that there is a Government commitment to strengthening the role of health services, noting that victim-survivors have indicated that healthcare workers are the professionals that they would be more likely to speak to about their experiences (Department of Health 2005; SafeLives n.d.). In 2014, the National Institute for Health and Care Excellence (NICE) published guidance to help health and social care commissioners and frontline practitioners whose work may bring them into contact with people who experience (or perpetrate) DVA. The aim of the guidance was to help identify, prevent and reduce domestic violence and abuse. The NICE guidance does acknowledge marginalised groups as people who experience abuse as there are brief sections on 'partner abuse among young people', 'abuse of older people' and 'honour'-based violence and forced marriage' (NICE 2014: 29–31). These are only scantily referenced, however, and the document identifies 'gaps in the evidence' pertaining to 'honour'-based violence, forced marriage, elder abuse, LGBT people and intimate partner violence among adolescents.

8.3 Lesbian, Gay, Bisexual, Trans and Queer Communities

As indicated in the Home Office's (2018) definition of DVA, and acknowledged by the World Health Organization (2017), DVA can be found in people's relationships irrespective of their gender and/or sexuality. As such, there is a sizeable body of global literature which explores the nature of DVA for lesbian, gay, bisexual, trans and queer (LGBTQ) communities. In terms of UK prevalence, using aggregated national survey data conducted between 2008 and 2011, Stonewall (Bachmann and Gooch 2018) claimed that one in four lesbian and bisexual women have experienced DVA in a relationship and almost half (49%) of all gay and bisexual men have experienced at least one incident of DVA from a family member or partner since the age of 16. There is limited research on how many trans or queer people experience DVA and existing studies have been conducted with small sample sizes. Nonetheless, the statistics available demonstrate that abuse experiences are common. For example, a small-scale study conducted in Scotland indicated that 80% of trans people have experienced some form of emotional, sexual, or physical abuse from a partner or ex-partner (Roch et al. 2010). In contrast, Rogers (2013, 2017) found that participants in her study were more likely to have experienced family violence than intimate partner abuse.

Whilst heterosexual and LGBTQ people might experience similar patterns of DVA, there are unique aspects of LGBTQ domestic violence and abuse. This includes:

- Threats of outing through disclosure of sexual orientation and gender identity to family, friends or work colleagues
- Threats of outing through disclosure of sexual orientation and gender identity to officials (for example, social workers for people with children)
- Undermining someone's sense of gender or sexual identity and exploiting a person's internalised negative self-beliefs
- Limiting or controlling access to spaces and networks that are helpful when coming to terms with gender and sexual identity and when coming out
- Controlling someone by convincing them that no-one would believe the abuse is real (exploiting heterosexist or heteronormative myths based on the 'public story')
- Manipulating victim-survivors into believing that abuse is a 'normal' part of same-sex relationships or pressuring victim-survivors into submission by minimalising abuse in the name of protecting the image of the LGBTQ community.

In addition, there are some trans-specific abuses which include withholding medication, preventing treatment or hiding gender signifiers (clothing, accessories, wigs) that are needed to express victim's gender identity or coercing someone into not pursuing medical treatment or gender reassignment. Identity abuse can occur when an abuser refuses to use somebody's preferred name, the correct pronouns or threatens to out a person by disclosing someone's trans history. An abuser might use derogatory names and use 'body shaming' tactics (being derisory or ridiculing a person's body image) to manipulate and control. It is likely that these behaviours are not uncommon as a small-scale survey ($n = 71$) found that almost half of respondents (46%) reported DVA that was transphobic in nature (Scottish Transgender Alliance 2008).

Box 8.1 Case Study: Sam

Sam, aged 36 years old, had identified as a trans male for 2 years and he had recently started to take hormones. Sam lived with his partner, Brian. They had been together for 14 years when Sam disclosed his trans identity. Sam and Brian had two children: Beccy (aged 10) and Britney (aged 8). After the children had started school Sam had found work in the local gym as a receptionist. Brian was home alone most days, unable to work having endured a back injury in his former job as an electrician. When they met Sam was 18 years old and Brian was 33. Sam said:

> Brian is older than me and I have always looked up to him. I didn't have many friends at school, and I grew up in care and so never felt that I had much family. With Brian, I got a, you know, the sense of being in a family and that someone loved me. I'd never felt that I belonged to a family or to someone.

When Sam first disclosed that he was trans, Brian's response was to accuse Sam of having an affair with a colleague from the gym. Sam described how she'd always thought that Brian was open-minded and their best friends, Simon and Jonny, were in a same-sex relationship. Sam described Brian's behaviour after he had come out:

> In the few months after I told Brian, he kept telling me to get to the doctors and that I obviously had something wrong with my head. One night we were sat watching the telly and it was about trans people. Brian got more and more angry. He grabbed my shirt and, right in my face, shouted 'you'll never do it. You're not a man. I'm a real man. You'll always be a woman.' He told me to stop this rubbish, or get out. He got up, didn't even look at me, and went upstairs. It came from nowhere. I was utterly shocked. So shocked, I couldn't speak.

Nothing further happened for a few months other than a few mean comments from Brian every now and then when he had too much to drink. In the last 6 months, however, Sam had experienced lots of emotional abuse. Sam felt that Brian was playing mind games as his clothes kept disappearing and Brian would come home with presents that Sam did not particularly like or that reflected his former female identity (such as a cup with 'best mom', or clothing/accessories that were feminine in style). In the past couple of months Brian had become sexually demanding. He was also becoming more and more controlling and resentful if Sam went out without him. As a result, he rarely left the house without Brian other than to take/collect the girls to school and when going to work.

Time to Reflect

You are a healthcare professional who met Sam at a clinic for a condition unrelated to his trans status and he disclosed abuse to you. What do you think would be an 'enabler' in terms of supporting Sam to access help to leave this abusive relationship?

Any combination of abuse dynamics and behaviours identified earlier can prevent someone from speaking out. Indeed, the barriers to help-seeking behaviour for people who belong to LGBTQ communities are multiple and for those people who have previously experienced or expect homo/bi/transphobic responses from support services and/or the criminal justice system, this can be a significant barrier to speaking out. SafeLives (2018) recently reported that just 2.5% of all victim-survivors accessing DVA services in England and Wales identify as LGBTQ. The reasons for this are complex and multiple but studies of DVA in LGBTQ communities have indicated that abuse is not always recognised as such, but considered to be 'just something that happened' or 'wrong but not a crime' (Roch et al. 2010: 5). This may be the power of the 'public story' in action.

Research internationally indicates high levels of LGBTQ DVA with a higher risk of DVA for LGBTQ individuals compared to their heterosexual peers (Langenderfer-Magruder et al. 2016). In the US, a large-scale survey undertaken each year found that the rate of reporting for DVA rose by almost 6% from 2032 reports in 2016 to 2144 reports in 2017 (NCAVP 2017). The survey also reported that the number of domestic homicides in 2017 was slightly higher to those recorded in 2016. Of the 16 domestic homicides, nine victims (56%) were men, five (31%) were women and one victim (6%) was a trans man (NCAVP 2017). In Australia, it is reported that LGBTQ individuals experience DVA at similar rates as for heterosexual people (Campo and Tayton 2015). Yet, reflecting the earlier discussion, in Australia there has been an invisibility of LGBTQ relationships in policy and practice responses and a lack of acknowledgement that intimate partner violence exists in these communities (Campo and Tayton 2015).

8.4 Men's Experiences of DVA

The majority of DVA research considers women's victimhood and the debate about whether violence perpetrated against women and men has the same meaning and impact is unrelenting (Morgan and Wells 2016). This debate is contentious as there are writers who argue fiercely that the two are not comparable as women's experiences are rooted to the enduring dynamics and outcomes of patriarchy and gender inequality; both permeate societies and affect women in wide-ranging aspects of personal life (Stark 2007; Corbally 2015). As such, gender inequality is structural and it is associated with men's desire for power and control; key elements in women's experiences of DVA. There is no doubt that men's use of DVA against women is a serious and damaging problem experienced by women across the globe (WHO 2017) but there is also a growing body of literature which details men's victimisation (Drijber et al. 2013; Corbally 2015; Morgan and Wells 2016). Whilst acknowledging these debates, and that DVA occurs for men in same-sex relationships, the focus here is on heterosexual men as victim-survivors when women are the perpetrators of abuse.

In terms of how men experience DVA, the existing evidence highlights that the abuse of men takes the same forms as for women in that it can be physical, sexual, psychological, financial and as coercive control. Abuse can be perpetrated by current or former partners. A study of 372 male victim-survivors in the Netherlands found that men reported that more than half (54%) of female perpetrators used an object during physical attacks (Drijber et al. 2013), a finding reported in other studies (Strauss and Gelles 1986). It was not, however, clear whether violence was one-way or bidirectional with violence alternating between partners. In his typology of DVA, Johnson (2008) terms this form of bidirectional abuse as situational couple violence. This occurs when conflict turns to aggression and then violence. Johnson argues that this form of DVA has gender symmetry in that both men and women will be perpetrators at similar rates.

There are studies which show significant impacts for men such as severe injuries (Nowinski and Bowen 2012) and behaviours which reflect intimate terrorism (Hines and Douglas 2010), another form of abuse named by Johnson (As discussed in Chap. 3). Intimate terrorism most likely represents a small proportion of all DVA but predominates among the cases of women that come to the attention of DVA services, the criminal justice system and other public agencies. Whilst men do experience intimate terrorism (Hines and Douglas 2010), the data are clear and illustrate that the primary perpetrators in heterosexual couples are men (Johnson 2008).

The work of Johnson and others, in this respect, bolsters the 'public story' (Donovan and Hester 2014) and this in turn can operate to marginalise men's victimhood in discussions of DVA. This can serve to restrict men's help-seeking for many reasons. On an individual level, reasons such as shame, embarrassment, the fear of ridicule or not being believed serve as significant barriers to seeking help (Barber 2008; Morgan and Wells 2016). Drijber et al.'s (2013) study in the Netherlands found that men were reluctant to report their abuse as they felt that services would not support them and that even if they attempted to report their experiences to the police that no action would be taken. Furthermore, Corbally (2015) observes that secondary victimisation through the responses of structures such as school, the police and court system is common for male victims.

8.5   Women with Learning Disabilities

Whilst there is a vast body of evidence illustrating the scale and nature of DVA in the general population, there is a much smaller body of research detailing the DVA of women with physical and sensory impairments (Thiara et al. 2011).

Moreover, evidence and scholarship highlighting DVA in the lives of women with learning disabilities are strikingly absent from policy and practice (McCarthy 2017a). This invisibility is illustrated in the annual census figures from Women's Aid Federation England (WAFE) as their annual census report for 2017–2018 found that only 2.6% of 18,895 service users, who were supported by 49 DVA services in England, identified as having a learning disability (Women's Aid 2019). What the existing evidence does show is that, similar to women with physical and sensory disabilities, women with learning disabilities are reportedly more susceptible to abusive relationships, but, as indicated by the Women's Aid census, have less access to DVA support and services (Hughes et al. 2012). In addition, women with learning disabilities are at a higher risk of more frequent and prolonged DVA than non-disabled women and disabled men (Brownridge et al. 2008; McCarthy et al. 2015). Women with learning disabilities are more likely to experience DVA as they do not receive adequate sex education, often lack the knowledge of what is appropriate within a relationship (McCarthy 2017b) and may be perceived as easy to manipulate and exploit. In addition, those with communication impairments are less able to report abusive behaviour to the appropriate agencies (Martin et al. 2006).

The types of DVA experienced by women with learning disabilities are similar to non-disabled women in that abuse can be physical, sexual, psychological and financial. In addition, in McCarthy et al.'s (2015) study, women with learning disabilities described how their abusers used their impairment to belittle and exploit, and coercive control was common. In relation to knowledge about abuse behaviours such as these, there are various sources of information created by, with and for people with learning disabilities which detail the nature and impact of abuse in general, but there is a dearth of practice guidance and appropriate tools for those working in health and social care in this regard. Additionally, research by Olsen et al. (2017) suggests that professionals lack the knowledge and confidence to assess and support people with learning disabilities who have experienced DVA. This was also the case for healthcare professionals as in McCarthy et al.'s study (2015), little or no action was taken unless women explicitly asked for help.

There are various barriers to accessing appropriate support for women with learning disabilities. Access to information is often lacking with information not available in easy-to-read formats. In McCarthy et al.'s (2015) study of 15 women with learning disabilities, 11 were unfamiliar with the word 'refuge' or did not know what help it could provide. Risk assessment tools, such as the DASH (domestic abuse, stalking and 'honour'-based violence) risk checklist are not appropriate for women with learning disabilities. The DASH tool is a generic risk identification checklist, but does not address the specificity of the person being assessed in terms of learning disability and would not, therefore, account for this as having any relevance in terms of presenting the situation; for example, in representing a risk factor.

8.6   Black and Ethnic Minority Communities

Domestic violence and abuse affects people from all communities and there is no evidence to suggest that women from black or minority ethnic (BME) or cultural minority groups are at any more at risk than others, but the form of abuse may vary. In some communities, for example, DVA might be perpetrated by extended family or community members. It might involve 'honour'-based abuse, child marriage, forced marriage or female genital mutilation. It is difficult to gain an accurate picture of the scale of DVA as many crimes of these types are hidden and go unreported (not unlike the other hard-to-reach communities discussed in this chapter). However, statistics collated by Women's Aid Federation England (WAFE) give some illustration. For example, the 2017–8 WAFE Annual Survey highlighted that of the total number of women accessing community-based services, were 'White British', the next two biggest categories were 'Asian/Asian British Pakistani' at 4.8% and 'Black/African/Caribbean/Black British African" at 4.2% (with 23.6% in total representing BME women) (Women's Aid 2019).

Like people who identify as LGBT or Q, people from BME communities are very likely to experience additional barriers to help-seeking meaning that they do not always get the help that they need. Racism can compound experiences or be used to execute control and manipulate using fear of a racist response to prevent help-seeking behaviour. This fear is inflated if a person does not have a secure immigration status in this country (for example, if they are seeking asylum). There are additional challenges for women who do not have a secure immigration status as they are therefore unlikely to be able to access the same levels of support if they do not have access to public funding (Anitha 2011; Dudley 2017). If the abuser is from a BME background, the victim-survivor might not want to speak out in order to protect them from institutional racism, particularly if this has underpinned a prior experience. The fear of rejection from family or communities can be strong and act as a barrier to help-seeking.

The pressure that forced marriage brings can mean that there are worries about blame and damaging the family honour. This 'honour'-based ideology is associated with many ethnic groups, including communities from the Arab countries, Asian and African sub-continents as well as Gypsy, Roma and Travelling communities; see the case study of Bridget in Box 8.2. Various cultural and religious beliefs and norms based on patriarchal notions can be deeply embedded in such communities. 'Honour'-based violence and forced marriage pose problems in terms of identification and belonging, and these have become potent issues in debates on multiculturalism, citizenship, community cohesion and identity (Gill 2013). Forced marriage, in particular, is complex as it is less well understood and often contested but, importantly, it brings attention to whether consent to marriage is 'free', 'full' and 'informed' and this way it illuminates forms of forced marriage such as marriage as slavery, child marriage, marriage of convenience, marriage to acquire nationality and undesirable marriage (United Nations 2012).

Time to Reflect
What are the barriers to leaving for Bridget? What would help Bridget to leave Michael? How could a healthcare professional facilitate support for Bridget?

Box 8.2 Case Study: Bridget

Bridget is 32 years old and from an Irish Travelling Community. She married Michael when she was 16 years old and they have six children aged between 6 months and 16 years old. Michael holds strict and rigid expectations which are directed towards Bridget and the children. The running of the household reflects Michael's traditional views which are underpinned by patriarchal notions about gender norms, family practices and the division of labour. These views are widely held within their community too. Bridget is a devout Catholic and takes the children to church on a regular basis. Bridget has experienced abuse (physical, sexual, financial and emotional) from Michael starting on the day after they were married. In the last 2 years, Michael has become more demanding sexually and has raped Bridget on several occasions. Bridget knows that Michael's upbringing had been harsh; he had experienced cold and cruel parenting from his father and his mother had died in childbirth when Michael was just a boy. Bridget feels sorry for Michael as he has no other family nor anyone else to show him love or care.

Bridget has one sister, Mary, but, at times, Bridget struggles to maintain contact as Michael does not like her being out of the house. In the last year Bridget has managed to maintain contact with Mary every month when Mary visits. Bridget speaks to other women in her community, but is not close to anyone (and certainly has not discussed Michael's behaviour, or their marriage with the other women). Bridget has attempted to leave Michael twice before, but returned due to a strong sense of duty; she takes her wedding vows seriously. Bridget was also worried that she and her children would be expelled from their community and that they would be left without a place to call home and without a community to belong to. She also returned as Michael had promised to change (but this lasted for a day or two before signs of abusive behaviour began to creep back into day-to-day life).

8.7   Intersectionality

It is worth drawing attention to the fact that most people do not experience the world from one social location or because of one characteristic, but rather different aspects of their identity and background impacts on life experience. Intersectionality is a concept which has been used to analyse how people's different social positions overlap (Crenshaw 1989) or how social divisions are connected (Anthias 2008). Intersectionality frameworks were developed by Black feminist scholarship; a body of work originating in the 1970s. This work drew attention to persisting inequalities and the marginalisation of Black women initially through highlighting the ways in which white feminists failed to understand and theorise the multiplicity and complexity of identity (Richardson and Monro 2012). Intersectional analysis has been used to explore DVA at the junctures of race, class and gender (Sokoloff and Dupont 2005).

Traditionally, intersectionality frameworks have been employed to explore social divisions based on the interlinking of these (race, class and gender) but this limited usage has been critiqued along with the tendency to apply intersectionality in a rigid, mechanistic way (Anthias 2008; Ahmed 2015) or opaquely (Hines 2011). It is more useful to think of axes of difference (Yuval-Davis 2006), a matrix of domination (Hill Collins 2000), or of identity and its relation to a dynamic process of positionality (Ahmed 2015; Rogers and Ahmed 2017). Notwithstanding, intersectionality frameworks are helpful in reminding us to consider that narratives of violence and abuse are often underpinned by multiple, not singular, aspects of a person's identity, background and lived experience.

8.8   Health and Well-Being Impacts

There are many health and well-being impacts that are crosscutting in terms of outcomes for people who are affected by DVA. For example, there are health, mental health, economic, cultural and social impacts and within each of these categories, there are many different consequences of abuse and maltreatment. Physical injury and trauma are not uncommon for survivors of DVA. For people considered to be from hard-to-reach communities, there can be additional impacts: for example, for BME women, their abuser might limit or control their access to medical appointments or medication impacting on their health primarily. The fear of retribution from the community can also cause considerable stress and anxiety. For trans people, their abusers might limit or hide the things they need to maintain their gender transitioning (hiding or destroying hormone medication for example) which can be psychologically distressing.

Time to Reflect
Can you think of other specific health and well-being impacts of DVA that might affect people from the hard-to-reach communities included in this chapter?

8.9   Best Practice with Hard-to-Reach Groups

Many things can inform best practice when working with victim-survivors of DVA (such as conceptual and practice-focused frameworks as well as specific models and techniques). Best practice can be reified in something as simple as person-centred communication which asks questions about the micro-level (everyday) factors which affect an individual: for example, the more practical issues such as financial arrangements or the responsibility of having a pet, for instance. This can include the recognition of the complexity of emotions (such as love, duty, shame, self-blame and guilt). It is important to consider a person's informal and formal social networks in terms of their extended family, community membership or relationships with employers, colleagues or agencies already involved with the family. Best practice with hard-to-reach groups, however, should also acknowledge macro-level factors such as institutional racism and structural inequalities. As the dynamics of abuse are inevitably entwined with power and control, it is imperative that our practice is mindful of this, and of the ways in which our engagement and intervention should seek to not reinforce the experiences of marginalisation and disempowerment.

Frameworks for practice, such as cultural competence and cultural humility, exist to support best practice with hard-to-reach groups. Effective engagement can rely on cultural competence which means that practitioners consider the social characteristics and backgrounds of victim-survivors (for example, gender, ethnicity, language, (dis) ability and other aspects of social location) (Birkenmaier et al. 2014). Before you can do this, you need to practice cultural humility which is the readiness to suspend what you know, or what you think you know, about a person using stereotypes and typecasting which are based on their culture, appearance or characteristics. Rather, what you learn about a person and their culture, background or identity evolves from what they express as being an important part of their sense of self and experiences of everyday life. There is another useful model that can underpin best practice with hard-to-reach groups and this is termed structural competence (Willging et al. 2019). A structural competency approach emerged in healthcare as a means of advancing the cultural competence model (which has been criticised for operating at a micro-level, recognising individual bias and prejudice only) to one which also embeds an acknowledgement of vulnerability and unequal outcomes as resulting from structural forces (which are much harder to break down) (Willging et al. 2019).

8.10   Summary

This chapter explored the global phenomenon of DVA. It has, however, departed from the 'public story' to discuss the issue from the perspective of different hard-to-reach groups including: LGBTQ populations; male victims; women with learning disabilities; and BME communities. Early in this chapter, it was argued that such groups have been hidden in much of the research, policy and practice on DVA, but that for each group there is a growing body of evidence to suggest that DVA is experienced at alarming rates. The chapter explored some of the barriers for hard-to-reach groups and provided case studies and reflective questions to help the reader to consider how healthcare practitioners can facilitate access to support, noting how it is reported that victim-survivors frequently state that they would rather disclose abuse experiences of healthcare practitioners than other professionals involved in their lives. This means that healthcare professionals are often best placed to help break down the barriers that hard-to-reach groups face in the context of DVA.

Summary Points
- As a healthcare professional you should be able to identify the additional barriers to recognising and naming their experiences as abuse for victim-survivors from hard-to-reach groups

- An appreciation of the additional barriers that prevent help-seeking and make it difficult to access appropriate support for victim-survivors from hard-to-reach groups
- Good practice in supporting victim-survivors from hard-to-reach groups includes a structural competency approach in order to consider individual experiences in the context of structural, systemic and institutional equalities and oppressions

8.11 Web Resources

- Barnados—Real Love Rocks. The online space all about raising awareness around child sexual exploitation and what a healthy and safe relationship is. https://www.barnardosrealloverocks.org.uk/
- Mankind is a confidential helpline for men escaping domestic violence. Website: www.mankind.org.uk. Telephone: 01823 334244.
- Galop's National LGBT Domestic Abuse Helpline is run by and for LGBT people and offers practical and emotional support to LGBT people experiencing domestic abuse. Website: www.galop.org.uk. Telephone: 0800 999 5428.
- The Forced Marriage Unit offers protection, advice and support to victims of forced marriage as well as information and practice guidelines for professionals. Website: https://www.gov.uk/guidance/forcedmarriage. Telephone: +44 (0) 207 008 0151. Email: fmu@fco.gov.uk and email for outreach work: fmuoutreach@fco.gov

References

Ahmed A (2015) Retiring to Spain: women's narratives of nostalgia, belonging and community. Policy Press, Bristol
Ahmed A, Rogers M (2016) Working with marginalised group: from policy to practice. Palgrave Macmillan, London
Anitha S (2011) Legislating gender inequalities: the nature and patterns of domestic violence experienced by South Asian women with insecure immigration status in the United Kingdom. Violence Against Women 17(10):1260–1285
Anthias F (2008) Thinking through the lens of translocation positionality: an intersectionality frame for understanding identity and belonging. Translocat Migr Soc Chang 4(1):5–20
Bachmann CL, Gooch B (2018) LGBT in Britain: trans report. Stonewall, London
Barber CF (2008) DV against men. Nurs Stand 22(51):35–39
Birkenmaier J, Berg-Weger M, Dewees MP (eds) (2014) The practice of generalist social work, 3rd edn. Routledge, London
Brownridge DA, Ristock J, Heibert-Murphy D (2008) The high risk of IPV against Canadian women with disabilities. Med Sci Monit 14:PH27–PH32
Campo M, Tayton S (2015) Intimate partner violence in lesbian, gay, bisexual, trans, intersex and queer communities: key issues. Australian Institute of Family Studies, Melbourne
Cook D (2002) Consultation, for a change? Engaging users and communities in the policy process. Soc Policy Adm 36(5):516–531
Corbally M (2015) Accounting for intimate partner violence: a biographical analysis of narrative strategies used by men experiencing IPV from their female partners. J Interpers Violence 30:3112–3132

Crenshaw K (1989) Demarginalizing the intersection of race and sex: a black feminist critique of antidiscrimination doctrine: feminist theory and antiracist politics. Univ Chic Leg Forum 140:138–167

Department of Health (2005) Responding to domestic abuse: a handbook for health professionals. Department of Health, London

Donovan C, Hester M (2014) Domestic violence and sexuality: what's love got to do with it? Policy Press, Bristol

Drijber BC, Reijnders UJL, Ceelen M (2013) Male victims of domestic violence. J Fam Violence 28:173–178

Dudley RG (2017) Domestic abuse and women with 'no recourse t public funds': the state's role in shaping and reinforcing coercive control. Fam Relatsh Soc 6(2):201–217

Flanagan SM, Hancock B (2010) 'Reaching the hard to reach' - lessons learned from the VCS (voluntary and community sector). A qualitative study. BMC Health Serv Res 10:92

Gill A (2013) Intersecting inequalities: implications for addressing violence against black and minority ethnic women in the United Kingdom. In: Lombard N, MacMillan L (eds) Violence against women: current theory and practice in domestic abuse, sexual violence and exploitation. Jessica Kingsley Publishers, London

Hill Collins P (2000) Black feminist thought: knowledge, consciousness, and the politics of empowerment, 2nd edn. Routledge, New York

Hines S (2011) Sexing gender; gendering: towards an intersectional analysis of transgender. In: Taylor Y, Hines S, Casey ME (eds) Theorizing intersectionality and sexuality. Palgrave Macmillan, Basingstoke

Hines DA, Douglas EM (2010) A closer look at men who sustain intimate terrorism by women. Partn Abus 1:286–313

Home Office (2016) Ending violence against women and girls: strategy 2016–2020. https://www.gov.uk/government/uploads/system/uploads/attachment_data/file/522166/VAWG_Strategy_FINAL_PUBLICATION_MASTER_vRB.PDF

Home Office (2018) Domestic violence and abuse: new definition. https://www.gov.uk/guidance/domestic-violence-and-abuse

Hughes K, Bellis MA, Jones L, Wood S, Bates G, Eckley L, McCoy E, Mikton C, Shakespeare T, Officer A (2012) Prevalence and risk of violence against adults with disabilities: a systematic review and meta-analysis of observational studies. Lancet 36(11):61851–61855

Johnson MP (2008) A typology of domestic violence: intimate terrorism, violence resistance and situational couple violence. Northwestern University Press, Boston

Langenderfer-Magruder L, Whifield DL, Walls NE, Kattari SK, Ramos D (2016) Experiences of intimate partner violence and subsequent police reporting among lesbian, gay, bisexual, transgender, and queer adults in Colorado: comparing rates of cisgender and transgender victimization. J Interpers Violence 31(5):855–871

Manjoo R (2015) Report of the Special Rapporteur on violence against women, its causes and consequences. United National Human Rights Council, Geneva

Martin SL, Ray N, Sotres-Alvarez D, Kupper LL, Moracco KE, Dickens A et al (2006) Physical and sexual assault of women with disabilities. Health Soc Care Community 14:284–293

McCarthy M (2017a) Learning disabilities and domestic abuse: an unspoken barrier. Safe Domestic Abuse Q (59):18–22

McCarthy M (2017b) 'What kind of abuse is him spitting in my food?': reflections on the similarities between disability hate crime, so-called 'mate' crime and domestic violence against women with intellectual disabilities. Disabil Soc 32(4):595–600

McCarthy M, Hunt S, Mine-Skillman K (2015) 'I know it was every week, but I can't be sure if it was everyday': domestic violence and women with learning disabilities. J Appl Res Intellect Disabil 29:1–14

Morgan W, Wells M (2016) 'It's deemed unmanly': men's experiences of intimate partner violence (IPV). J Forensic Psychiatry Psychol 27(3):404–418

NCAVP (2017) Lesbian, gay, bisexual, transgender, queer and hiv-affected hate and intimate partner violence in 2017: a report from the national coalition of anti-violence programs. NCAVP, New York

NICE (2014) Domestic violence and abuse: how health services, social care and the organisations they work with can respond effectively. NICE, London

Nowinski SN, Bowen E (2012) Partner violence against heterosexual and gay men: prevalence and correlates. Aggress Violent Behav 17:36–52

Olsen A, Majeed-Ariss R, Teniola S, White C (2017) Improving service responses for people with learning disabilities who have been sexually assaulted: an audit of forensic services. Br J Learn Disabil 45(4):238–245

Richardson D, Monro S (2012) Sexuality, equality and diversity. Palgrave Macmillan, London

Roch A, Ritchie G, Morton J (2010) Transgender people's experiences of domestic abuse. LGBT Youth Scotland and the Equality Network, Scotland

Rogers M (2013) TransForming practice: trans people's experiences of domestic abuse. PhD Thesis, University of Sheffield, Sheffield

Rogers M (2016) Funding cuts could leave victims of domestic violence with nowhere to go, the conversation, 22 June 2016. https://theconversation.com/funding-cuts-could-leave-victims-of-domestic-violence-with-nowhere-to-go-61177

Rogers M (2017) Transphobic 'honour'-based abuse: a conceptual tool. Sociology 51(2):225–240

Rogers M, Ahmed A (2017) Interrogating trans and sexual identities through the conceptual lens of translocational positionality. Sociol Res Online 22(1). https://doi.org/10.1016/j.adolescence.2015.11.003. http://www.socresonline.org.uk/22/1/contents.html

SafeLives (2018) Free to be safe: LGBT people experiencing domestic abuse. SafeLives, Bristol

SafeLives (n.d.) A Cry for Health Why we must invest in domestic abuse services in hospitals. http://safelives.org.uk/cry-for-health. Accessed 22 March 2019

Scottish Transgender Alliance (2008) Transgender experiences in Scotland. http://www.scottish-trans.org/Uploads/Resources/staexperiencessummary03082.pdf. Accessed 13 Jan 2015

Sokoloff HJ, Dupont I (2005) Domestic violence at the intersections of race, class and gender. Violence Against Women 11(1):38–64

Stark E (2007) Coercive control: how men entrap women in personal life. Oxford University Press, New York

Strauss MA, Gelles RJ (1986) Societal change and change in family violence from 1975 to 1985 as revealed by two national surveys. J Marriage Fam 48:465–479

Thiara RK, Hague G, Mullender A (2011) Losing out on both counts: disabled women and domestic violence. Disabil Soc 26:757–771

United Nations (2012) Core elements of legislation on forced marriage and child marriage. http://www.endvawnow.org/en/articles/611-core-elements-of-legislation-on-forced-and-child-marriage-.html?next=612

WHO (2017) Violence against women: key facts. http://www.who.int/en/news-room/fact-sheets/detail/violence-against-women. Accessed 26 Mar 2019

Wilkerson JM, Iantaffi A, Grey JA, Bockting WO (2014) Recommendations for internet-based qualitative health research with hard-to-reach populations. Qual Health Res 24(4):561–574

Willging C, Gunderson L, Shattuck D, Sturm R, Lawyer A, Crandall C (2019) Structural competency in emergency medicine services for transgender and gender non-conforming patients. Soc Sci Med 222:67–75

Women's Aid (2019) The domestic abuse report 2019: the annual audit. Women's Aid, Bristol

Yuval-Davis N (2006) Intersectionality and feminist politics. Eur J Women's Stud 13(3):193–201

Domestic Violence and Abuse and Working with Other Agencies

9

Julie McGarry and Parveen Ali

9.1 Introduction

Domestic violence and abuse is a complex issue that needs sensitive handling by a range of health and social care professionals. (National Institute for Clinical Care Excellence (NICE) 2014).

Domestic violence and abuse (DVA) is inherently complex and supporting DVA victim-survivors requires coordinated and wide efforts across a range of roles within and across organisations. In previous chapters, we have highlighted the profound and far-reaching impact of DVA on the lives and health of all those who experience DVA. We have also identified that DVA exerts a significant and detrimental impact on the lives and health of those who experience abuse, and on wider family members and especially children whether or not they directly witness or experience DVA. In the UK, as elsewhere, there has been a growing recognition of the key role that healthcare professionals play in responding to those who are experiencing or have experienced abuse. As healthcare organisations can be transit places for those accessing services, healthcare professionals—including doctors, nurses, midwives and others are well placed to—identify those experiencing DVA (or at risk of experiencing DVA), deal with their health concerns and finally refer them to appropriate

J. McGarry (✉)
School of Health Sciences, The University of Nottingham, Queen's Medical Centre, Nottingham, UK
e-mail: Julie.McGarry@nottingham.ac.uk; https://institutemh.org.uk/research/centre-for-social-futures/projects/349-research-area-domestic-violence-and-abuse

P. Ali
School of Health Sciences, The University of Sheffield, Sheffield, UK
e-mail: parveen.ali@sheffield.ac.uk

© Springer Nature Switzerland AG 2020
P. Ali, J. McGarry (eds.), *Domestic Violence in Health Contexts: A Guide for Healthcare Professions*, https://doi.org/10.1007/978-3-030-29361-1_9

services in or around the community where they (patients) live and can be better supported for their needs. In addition, as noted above (NICE 2014), there has been an increasing acknowledgment of the importance for professionals and agencies to work together to facilitate effective identification of DVA and support for victim-survivors and families (NICE 2014, 2016). The aim of this chapter, therefore, is to consider the range of professionals and wider agencies and services who may have the potential to work alongside healthcare professionals in supporting victim-survivors of DVA and, where appropriate, family members. Using a real life example from a Serious Case Review (SCR) and a report entitled *Breaking Down the Barriers* (2019) we will explore the inherent complexities of multi-agency working and the enablers and barriers to working collaboratively across professional and disciplinary boundaries.

Time to Reflect
You are providing services to a victim-survivor of DVA and now must think about referral to other agencies. Take a moment to consider which agencies and professionals may need to be involved in supporting and/or providing services to a victim-survivor of DVA.

9.2 Which Agencies and Services Provide Support for Victim-Survivors of DVA?

DVA has harmful impacts for individuals, families and relationships. It affects health, well-being and education of children witnessing or experiencing abuse. It affects the economy, businesses and employers in the community where victim-survivors or perpetrators work. It increases demands of housing and results in other health and social care needs. All these service providers and agencies are affected and often deal with the same issue in divergent ways, with different interventions and different outcomes. At the same time, it is important to remember that there are many different healthcare professionals as part of multidisciplinary team who should be involved when providing services to DVA victim-survivors and families.

Time to Reflect
Make a list of different healthcare professionals who make up the multidisciplinary team in your organisation and who could be involved in the provision of services for those who have experienced DVA (this will vary depending upon where you are based).

It will also be useful for you to take a moment to consider the wide range of professionals, provider services and specialist agencies who may be involved in supporting victim-survivors of DVA. These include—but are not limited to—primary and secondary health care services, mental health services, sexual violence services, social care, criminal justice agencies, the police, probation, youth justice, substance misuse, specialist DVA agencies, children's services, housing services and education (Fig. 9.1). The list is not exhaustive, but highlights the range and

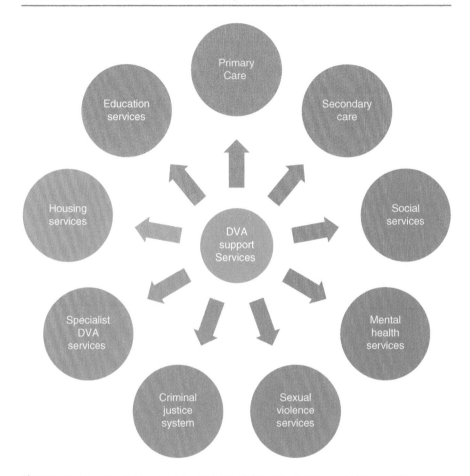

Fig. 9.1 Various agencies involved in provision of domestic violence and abuser services

diversity of services and organisations that may be involved with victim-survivors of DVA and families–and the potential issues in relation to effective cross-agency working. You may have experiences from your own practice that you can draw on to add to the list.

Involvement of various agencies in the providing support is known as a 'multi-agency response'. The concept of multi-agency response was initially known as 'the coordinated community response' (CCR) in Duluth, Minnesota, Untied States. The idea was that, having a coordinated response from different local services would help to reduce DVA, keep victims and children safe and hold perpetrators account-able for their abusive behaviour and help to improve service provision (Hague and Bridge 2008). Evidence suggests that working in a multi-agency partnership is the most effective way to respond to DVA at an operational and strategic level. Whilst victim-survivors can tell a lot about their experiences, they may not be in an optimal position (DVA experiences may hamper their ability to analyse situation effectively and objectively although of course this is individual specific) to assess accurately the risk of harm in their situation and the need for additional support. Healthcare professionals must take this into account and may actively seek additional information from the multi-agency network and work with them to ensure victim-survivors and their dependent children are safeguarded.

The level of multiple engagement with services or agencies/organisations may be dependent on the circumstances or complexity of each individual case and its surrounding situation and the availability of services in the local area. To place this into context we have drawn on the 2019 Report *Breaking Down the Barriers* (Against Violence and Abuse 2019) which presents the findings of a national commission on domestic and sexual violence and multiple disadvantage among women. The aims of this report were, essentially: to examine the links between domestic and sexual violence and multiple disadvantage (and to consider the impact of intersectionality within this, for example, accounting for socioeconomic position); to gather the experiences of women and provision of services; and to collate evidence and identify ways forward. The rationale for the commission was that women who have experienced DVA also experience high rates of poverty, homelessness and mental ill-health. The report highlighted that many women who are in contact with the criminal justice system have experienced domestic or sexual violence, further emphasising the potential overlaying of complexity–and involvement of services–surrounding DVA. In developing the background for the report, peer researchers (i.e. those with lived experience) worked with women participants to collaboratively develop a model of what multiple disadvantage (Fig. 9.2) meant for them.

The model above illustrates several common threads (in the three corners of the triangle) for the women—mental ill-health, substance use and domestic and sexual violence. The centre of the model highlights the outcomes that women faced–and as you can see, these clearly resonate with our list of potential services and agencies above–and again highlights the far-reaching impact and complexity of DVA. The outer periphery of the model represents how women felt caught in the stigma which 'labelled them as problematic, complex, chaotic, damaged or harmed' (p. 7).

Several key themes and recommendations emerged from the report, which is available in full at the end of the chapter and we would recommend accessing this for a more detailed account of the background and recommendations. The report highlighted, for example, that women who experience multiple disadvantage do not typically access specialist DVA services, but rather present at multiple services (including healthcare) various times. However, health services, among other services, are often poorly prepared to support women and/or work across organisational boundaries. Different services do not always communicate with each other, resulting in lack of sharing information. Consequently, the victim-survivor must provide their information, including details of their abusive experiences repeatedly to different people in different organisations. Recalling experiencing can itself be traumatic for victim-survivors and consequently may deter them from accessing support. Several suggestions to address this deficit were made in the report and included 'one stop shops' and co-location of professionals and services. The report also highlighted the absence of a coherent and 'joined up' strategy for working across agencies and organisations and the need for this to be addressed on a national

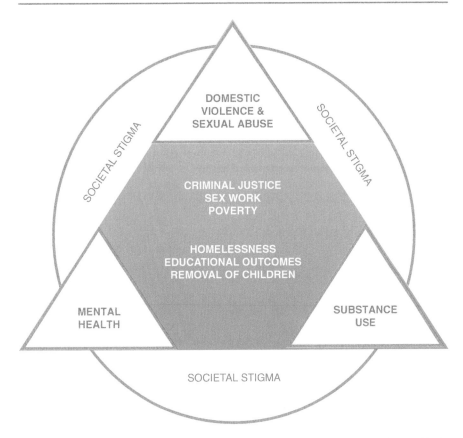

Fig. 9.2 Multiple disadvantage taken from *Breaking Down the Barriers* and reproduced with the kind permission of AVA (Against Violence and Abuse)

level. This fact is relevant in the context of the UK, and in any country and health and social care system in the world.

We have provided a very brief overview of *Breaking Down the Barriers* (2019) but in so-doing and in directing you to the report, hope that you will gain a broader insight into the multilayered phenomenon of DVA and consider the list that we provided originally within the context of the model of multiple disadvantage in Fig. 9.1. In addition, there could be other professionals and organisations that may need to be involved in the provision of appropriate services such as interpretation services or perpetrator services.

9.3 Why Is Multi-agency Working Important?

Having considered the multi-faceted and complex issues surrounding DVA and the many different agencies who may be involved, we now turn to consider the question of why multi-agency working is so important in this context and we will do this by

Box 9.1 Overview of SCR, SAR and DHR

Serious Case Reviews (SCRs):

These relate to serious cases where abuse or neglect of a child is known or suspected and the child has died or the child has been seriously harmed and there is cause for concern as to the way in which the local authority, their Board partners or other relevant persons have worked together to safeguard the child (Working Together to Safeguard Children 2015).

Over the forthcoming year, these reviews will be replaced by Child Safeguarding Practice Reviews conducted under the new safeguarding partnership arrangements (Working Together to Safeguard Children 2018). Part of the new process is to complete the research for potential reviews using a rapid review process.

Safeguarding Adult Reviews (SARs):

An SAR must be conducted where "there is reasonable cause for concern about how the Safeguarding Adults Board, members of it or others worked together to safeguard the adult and death or serious harm arose from actual or suspected abuse." (Care Act 2014) A review may also be commissioned in other circumstances where it is felt one would be useful, including learning from 'near misses'.

Domestic Homicide Reviews (DHRs):

A DHR must be conducted where the death of a person aged 16 or over has, or appears to have, resulted from violence, abuse or neglect by a person to whom the victim was related or with whom the victim was or had been in an intimate personal relationship, or a member of the same household. This definition has been extended to include deaths by suicide where domestic violence has been identified.

exploring a real life Serious Case Review (SCR) involving an older couple, Mr. and Mrs. A. This SCR has been widely reported in the media. You may see the term SCR used, although, as noted in Box 9.1, Safeguarding Adults Review (SAR) is more usual. We have also included Domestic Homicide Review (DHR) and have provided an explanation of the different types of review in Box 9.1. In this case the SCR was commissioned in relation to the involvement of all agencies with Mr. and Mrs. A. Both Mr. and Mrs. A were admitted to hospital on the same day following an incident at their home. Mrs. A died shortly after her admission to hospital and Mr. A died in hospital 18 days later.

9.4 Case Study: Mr. and Mrs. A

Mr. and Mrs. A had been married for 56 years at the time of Mrs. A's death. They had, until relatively recently, little support from outside agencies other than primary care services. Mr. and Mrs. A were registered at different general practitioner (GP) practices. Mrs. A was deemed to have the capacity to make her own decisions–both by her family and outside agencies. Mrs. A experienced several health issues, but these were managed by the primary health care team. Mrs. A walked with the aid of a walking stick, but was otherwise mobile. Mr. A was also deemed to have capacity by the professionals involved in his care (the exception to this was the attending police officers who, after discussion with Mrs. A, concluded that Mr. A was experiencing cognitive impairment related to age). Mr. A was increasingly limited in his mobility–he had experienced several falls–but was able to mobilise within the home. Mr. and Mrs. A were clear that they did not want any support from social care or any other intervention except in the event of a crisis.

In the period 2006–2010 prior to death, there were six recorded references to DVA and all but one were verbal in nature. Four reports were made to Mrs. A's GP and two to social services–who observed one incident of verbal abuse by Mrs. A to her husband. Mrs. A's GP did not refer to any outside agency. In 2010, there was a further nine separate incidents of physical abuse reported by Mrs. A–some were reported to more than one agency. All agencies responded promptly and were concerned for Mrs. A's safety. Mrs. A was given options and offers of additional help in the home. Mrs. A would not allow social services to speak to her son or daughter. When Mrs. A dialled '999' (the UK police emergency line) each incident was treated as a 'stand-alone' incident. Mrs. A explained Mr. A's behaviour as part of his deteriorating mental health. Mr. A was interviewed by police during which he stated that his wife 'sometimes abused him, including with her nails'. Whilst a referral was made to the Multi Agency Risk Assessment Conference (MARAC),[1] Mr. A's disclosure was not reported at the meeting. Mr. A was seen by police officers during their responses to calls, but his views were not elicited due to the beliefs regarding cognitive impairment. During admission to hospital Mr. A reported that he was being abused by his wife–this was taken seriously by ambulance, hospital staff and social services staff. However, the police were not informed, and Mr. A wanted to go home. Moreover, on admission to hospital Mr. A was visibly 'thin' and was hungry (although having spent time on the floor following a fall was felt to account for the hunger). On discharge the care package that had been arranged was swiftly cancelled by Mr. and Mrs. A. Sometime afterwards, Mrs. A was admitted to hospital following a '999' call and died later that day.

---

[1] A MARAC is a regular local meeting to discuss how to help victims at high risk of murder or serious harm. In this meeting various professionals involved in provision of services to victim-survivor, including a domestic abuse specialist (IDVA), police, children's social services, health and other relevant agencies come together to discuss this issue. Each case is reviewed and details of particular victim-survivor, their children, other family members, perpetrator and other contextual information is shared in the group so all involved can analyse the situation appropriately before coming to any conclusion and making decisions. The meeting is confidential. For further details of the composition and function of a MARAC please see http://www.safelives.org.uk/practice-support/resources-marac-meetings

Time to Reflect

Having read the case study above, we would like you to consider the following questions:

- **What are your initial thoughts about the case? For example, do you think that there were 'missed opportunities' for different organisations to liaise with each other?**
- **How do you think that the professionals and services viewed Mr. and Mrs. A? Do you think for example, that they held any assumptions based on age?**
- **What do you think was the role of healthcare professionals in the case study?**
- **How do you think Mr. and Mrs. A's case could have been approached differently?**

9.5   'Lessons Learned': Our Reflections on the Case Study

This was a very difficult, and—as so often with DVA—a complex case. In the SCR, the opportunities that were missed by several key agencies were highlighted as central. These largely centred on a lack of communication between agencies and the way the reported instances of DVA or abuse were treated separately—rather than forming a part of a more complete picture of the home situation. The age of Mr. and Mrs. A may also have been a factor in terms of a poor understanding among professionals of DVA as occurring in later life and the associated level of risk and/or other possible vulnerabilities. Although the services involved did undertake risk assessments and, on the whole, appropriate referrals were made (for example, to MARAC)—again, these were undertaken by different organisations as separate entities.

In terms of lessons learned, some of the themes of this case study have been identified in recent publications. In *Standing Together against Domestic Violence: A Guide to Effective Domestic Violence Partnerships* (2013) a summary of key lessons which occur repeatedly within Domestic Homicide Reviews (DHRs) are listed below and these include: a lack of adherence to policies and practices (e.g. on risk assessment); where policies are followed, they sometimes replace professional judgement and, therefore, negate the expertise of the worker; not understanding the dynamic of DVA (e.g. escalation, manipulation by the perpetrator, victim behaviour); inadequate information sharing; inadequate support for those at standard and medium risk; lack of DVA training; lack of coordination among partner agencies; limited understanding of other factors affecting DVA (multiple disadvantage A: DV/substance misuse/mental health); absence of routine DVA enquiry; under resourced provision of specialist DVA services and problematic commissioning (e.g. poor quality of services) (Standing together against domestic violence, 2013).

Multi-agency working is a central issue that was highlighted in the case of Mr. and Mrs. A, a feature of *Breaking Down the Barriers* (2019), and highlighted above in *Standing Together against Domestic Violence: A Guide to Effective Domestic Violence Partnerships* (2013). There are more general issues associated with multi-agency working and these are summarised next.

9.6 Challenges Associated with Multi-agency Working

Highlighted in this chapter so far, is that collaborative or multi-agency working has its own challenges (Haas et al. 2011; Stanley et al. 2011). Fundamentally, different agencies and service provider have different organisational missions, visions, values, aims and objectives (Hester 2011). They have different targets and may also have different rules, regulations and working mechanisms. This makes it difficult for professionals in these agencies to work together at the same pace. There could also be a lack of understanding of the role and responsibilities of staff and the language used by individuals and organisations could be different leading to issues in working together. A good example to elaborate this is the difference in the language, definitions and labels used to refer to the victim-survivor with various labels in operation including 'victim' (criminal justice system), 'survivor' (women-centred organisation), 'patient' (healthcare services), 'tenant' (housing services) and 'service user'(welfare agencies) and 'customer' (adults social care). This highlights the complexities of working in multi-agency contexts (Robbins et al. 2014). Various agencies use different tools and instruments to asses and report DVA risk and data gathered by different agencies is not comparable due to variations in the type of data collected, ways it is recorded, data storage and lack or data portability mechanisms. There may also be differences in understanding of what constitute DVA and its impact among different organisations (Peckover et al. 2013). High staff turnover in organisations is also another barrier and affects communication as it takes time for people to develop trusting relationships (Haas et al. 2011).

In the final section of this chapter, we consider how healthcare professionals, alongside other agencies can develop effective partnerships and professional working practice.

9.7 What Constitutes a Successful Partnership in the Context of Multi-Agency Working?

As Ofsted and Stanley (2018) highlights, an understanding of the challenges of multi-agency working can help to identify components of successful multi-agency partnership and this section aims to explore these components (Fig. 9.3). The importance of leadership for any group and organisation cannot be underestimated. For an effective multi-agency partnership, it is essential that all partners have a clear and shared vision, clearly articulated and agreed goals, aims and objectives. It is equally important that the staff in all organisations are aware of the vision, mission and goals of the partnership and have had the opportunity to clarify any misconceptions or questions.

For any services, including multi-agency partnerships, to work effectively, it is important to understand the needs from the perspective various stakeholders including service users as well as frontline practitioners providing services. Such an understanding may help identify concerns and issues affecting the provision of services and, thereby, help set priorities for the services. For instance, an understanding

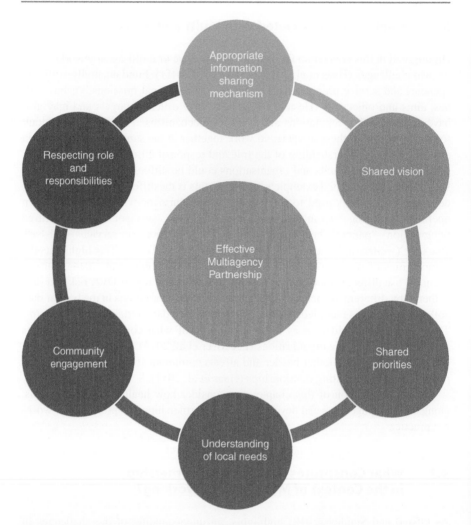

Fig. 9.3 Components of successful multi-agency partnership working

of current practices of healthcare professionals when dealing with DVA victim-survivors may identify lack of confidence among healthcare professionals with regards to asking appropriate questions and referring victim-survivors to appropriate services (Refer to Chap. 4). This knowledge can then be used to develop appropriate education and training resources to meet the needs of the healthcare professionals and to enhance their ability to identify and respond to DVA. Knowing such needs can help multi-agency to set up priorities effectively and to develop clear and SMART plans to meet those priorities. The staff in every agency in the partnership needs to be able to articulate reasons for the priorities and how they are going to work together to meet those priorities.

It is essential to use a joined-up approach, where various agencies are working together in order to smartly and effectively provide services. Such an approach may not seem different on the surface, but for victim-survivors and their children it can be beneficial as there will be less duplication of assessment, and provision of services would be integrated and efficient. An understanding and clarity of roles of various professionals working in the multi-agency context is very important. Professionals in different organisations and diverse disciplines bring different but complementary expertise. For example, the expertise, knowledge and skills of a practice nurse will be completely different from those of a social worker. Similarly, a police officer brings a very different set of experience and knowledge, than a domestic abuse advisor.

Appropriate and timely information sharing is very important. There should be clear mechanisms and protocols for sharing information—between agencies—and these should be promoted and monitored by management and supported by compatible IT (information technology) systems (NICE 2014). Effective information sharing relies on open communication and collaboration and facilitate the use of a common language among various professionals. Provision of shared training events for various professionals is also a good strategy to bring people in one place to facilitate the development of a shared language and understanding of information sharing as integral in the response to DVA.

Finally, the importance of monitoring, evaluation and auditing cannot be underestimated as it will help in identifying strengths, weaknesses, opportunities and challenges for the multi-agency partnership. Areas of improvements identified through such activities should be considered learning and improvement opportunities in which views of victim-survivors and all other stakeholders should be sought and incorporated.

9.8   Principles of Multi-agency Agency Working

To ensure successful partnership, certain principles can be developed and agreed on by different agencies working together. The points listed below can help professionals and organisations to draw and agree on certain principles that all agencies working together should adhere to:

- Understand that without effective prevention and early intervention DVA often escalates in severity and, therefore, it is important to make every effort to identify and support adult and child victims earlier.
- Prioritise safety of the victim-survivors and their children when considering interventions and acting immediately on disclosure of risk of harm.
- Data about all incidents of DVA should be recorded, analysed and shared with management of agencies working together regularly and appropriately.
- At the initial engagement with the services, informed consent of the victim-survivor should be gained to ensure information between agencies can be shared, when required, without unnecessary delay.
- Develop effective working relationships with specialist agencies and make appropriate representation and contribution to discussions in various forums, meetings and conferences when required.

- Work cooperatively to provide a supportive and enabling environment which encourages people to report DVA to police and other professionals and agencies.
- Respect confidentiality and privacy wherever possible and understand the risks associated with information sharing in the context of DVA.
- Develop and adhere to shared policies and procedures to guide information sharing between different organisations.
- Use a multi-agency and collaborative approach in holding perpetrators accountable for their actions.
- Ensure that perpetrators are known by appropriate and required agencies to ensure safety of the victim-survivor and that perpetrators may also be referred to appropriate services.
- Ensure that victim-survivors are treated with respect and dignity. By listening to them and believing their experiences and assuring them that they are never to blame.
- Empower DVA victim-survivors to make well-informed choices and decisions for themselves, wherever possible. Do not make decisions for them without their involvement.
- Work together to respect the rights of the family to stay as a family when working with them as much as possible.
- Ensure that services are sensitive to the diverse need of the victim-survivors considering their age, disability, gender, race or ethnicity, religion or belief, sexual orientation, but recognise that such differences are not used as an excuse for accepting or perpetrating DVA or other harmful practices.
- Acknowledge the impact of wider socioeconomic factors (low income, low literacy or numeracy skills, isolation or caring responsibilities) on DVA and ensure that appropriate support and services are available for those requiring support (for example with jobs, housing).
- Recognise additional barriers affecting access, availability and acceptability of services for victim-survivors of DVA (for example, women from minority ethnic background; those with disabilities; those with no recourse to funds or issues with migration status).
- Recognise that victim-survivors and their children are most at risk when attempting to leave an abusive relationship or seeking help.

9.9   Summary

In this chapter, we have sought to provide you with an overview of the different agencies and approaches that may be involved with supporting those who have experienced DVA alongside wider family members. We have also examined some of the issues and considerations when working within and across organisations. We also signpost the reader to several resources to support professional development and reflection.

Summary Points
- Healthcare professionals have a responsibility to identify, support and refer victim-survivors of DVA to relevant agencies and organisations.

- Effective responses to DVA require a coordinated approach across agencies and organisations.
- Communication is crucial in this process and healthcare professionals need to ensure that they are aware of the referral pathways and processes for victim-survivors of DVA.

Acknowledgements We would like to thank Hannah Hogg, Safeguarding Lead (Corporate). Nottinghamshire Healthcare NHS Foundation Trust for providing the text for Box 9.1 in this chapter.

Web Resources

https://avaproject.org.uk/breaking-down-the-barriers-findings-of-the-national-commission-on-domestic-and-sexual-violence-and-multiple-disadvantage/
IRIS website: http://www.irisdomesticviolence.org.uk/iris/

References

AVA (2019) Breaking down the barriers. https://avaproject.org.uk/wp/wp-content/uploads/2019/02/Breaking-down-the-Barriers-full-report-.pdf
Hague G, Bridge S (2008) Inching forward on domestic violence: the 'co-ordinated community response' and putting it into practice in Cheshire. J Gend Stud 17(3):185–199
Haas SM, Bauer-Leffler S, Turley E (2011) Evaluation of cross-disciplinary training on the co-occurrence of domestic violence and child victimization: overcoming barriers to collaboration. J Health Hum Serv Adm 34:352–386
Hester M (2011) The three planet model: towards an understanding of contradictions in approaches to women and children's safety in contexts of domestic violence. Br J Soc Work 41(5):837–853. https://doi.org/10.1093/bjsw/bcr095
National Institute of Clinical Excellence (2014) Domestic violence and abuse: multi-agency working. Public health guideline [PH50]. https://www.nice.org.uk/guidance/ph50
NICE (2016). Domestic violence and abuse NICE quality standard [QS116]. National Institute of Health and Care Excellence. https://www.nice.org.uk/guidance/qs116
Peckover S, Golding B, Cooling P (2013) Multi-agency working in domestic abuse and safeguarding children. https://www.centreforwelfarereform.org/uploads/attachment/369/multi-agency-working-in-domestic-abuse-and-safeguarding-children.pdf
Robbins R, McLaughlin H, Banks C, Bellamy C, Thackray D (2014) Domestic violence and multi-agency risk assessment conferences (MARACs): a scoping review. J Adult Prot 16(6):389–398
Stanley N, Miller P, Foster HR, Thomson G (2011) Children's experiences of domestic violence: developing an integrated response from police and child protection services. J Interpers Violence 26(12):2372–2391
Ofsted, Stanley Y (2018) Social care commentary: multi-agency safeguarding arrangements. https://www.gov.uk/government/speeches/social-care-commentary-multi-agency-safeguarding-arrangements

Refection and Implications for Healthcare Practice

10

Julie McGarry and Parveen Ali

10.1 Introduction

As we have identified throughout this book, DVA is an inherently complex phenomenon and is multi-factorial. It is not defined by the parameters of age, ethnicity or social class, but rather can be experienced and can affect almost everyone. We also know that DVA has both immediate and long-term consequences for health and well-being and that this includes physical as well as mental health. We have also highlighted that the impact of DVA can extend beyond those directly experiencing abuse, affecting other family members and especially children.

As we have highlighted in previous chapters, those who have experienced DVA may present to a number of healthcare settings, including Emergency Departments (ED) or primary care. However, those who have experienced DVA may in fact present to any and all areas of healthcare provision. Healthcare professionals, therefore, are in a pivotal position to ask about DVA and to support individuals following disclosure. While identification and support following disclosure are now part of the remit of a healthcare professional, many feel uncomfortable or ill-prepared to undertake this work (Ali and McGarry 2018). In this chapter, we explore some of the key practical considerations for healthcare professionals within the context of

J. McGarry (✉)
School of Health Sciences, The University of Nottingham, Queen's Medical Centre, Nottingham, UK
e-mail: Julie.McGarry@nottingham.ac.uk; https://institutemh.org.uk/research/centre-for-social-futures/projects/349-research-area-domestic-violence-and-abuse

P. Ali
School of Health Sciences, The University of Sheffield, Sheffield, UK
e-mail: Parveen.ali@sheffield.ac.uk

© Springer Nature Switzerland AG 2020

137

P. Ali, J. McGarry (eds.), *Domestic Violence in Health Contexts: A Guide for Healthcare Professions*, https://doi.org/10.1007/978-3-030-29361-1_10

their everyday work. We also consider the implications for further professional development and signpost the reader to relevant resources to support knowledge acquisition and practice development.

10.2   How and Where to Ask About DVA?

We know that healthcare professionals are in a key position to identify DVA and to refer victim-survivors to appropriate services. For example, in a study of 2500 women accessing DVA services almost 50% highlighted that prior to receiving specialist help they had attended a General Practitioner (GP) appointment, on average of just over five times, and one in five had attended the Emergency Department (ED) as a result of their abuse (Safe Lives 2012).

Within the literature and research in this field, healthcare professionals have often stated that they are reticent about asking patients or clients about DVA even where they suspect abuse is occurring. There may be a number of reasons for this reluctance to enquire about DVA, including fear of offending, lack of opportunity, associated time constraints if disclosure is made, lack of knowledge of where to refer and concerns regarding patient or client safety (Ahmad et al. 2017).

Why so many healthcare professionals may feel reticent about asking a patient or client about DVA is that they may not feel that they have the skills or confidence to do so. However, the evidence suggests that patients and clients are not offended when asked about DVA—and actually for those who have experienced DVA this may be the first opportunity for them to disclose. Safety, however, is paramount. Healthcare professionals need to ensure that they can speak with patients or clients in a private setting. Healthcare professionals also need to be cognisant of the need to ensure professional interpreter services where such services are required (this is discussed in greater detail in the Department of Health Resource below).

In the next section, we present some of the practical considerations that we would ask you to think about within your own area of practice.

10.3   Preparation and Awareness

We have already explored the important role healthcare professionals have in identifying and managing DVA. First step in this regard is being able to understand the possible causes, risk factors, manifestations and impact of DVA. Knowing about these aspects and the specific contexts in which DVA happens can be very useful in understanding the individual needs of victim-survivors. Appropriate training and education is necessary. Specifically, practitioners need to have a good understanding of their role and responsibilities, local policies and procedures and referral pathways (Ahmad et al. 2017). There are some examples of intervention developed to enhance the confidence and competence of healthcare professionals in identification, management and referral of victims-survivors of DVA such as the initiative IRIS (Identification and Referral to Improve Safety) in England (Bradbury-Jones et al. 2017). IRIS was developed and has since been tested successfully within the primary care setting in the UK (Feder et al. 2011). IRIS was designed initially to provide training and advocacy support for GPs and practice teams in the primary care setting in the identification, response and referral to specialist DVA advocacy support (Malpass et al. 2014). Following evaluation (Feder et al. 2011) IRIS has been commissioned as a service model across a number of regions in the UK (McGarry et al. 2019). We will now look at points to be considered in clinical practice.

10.4 Practical Points in Identification

In some areas of practice, there are particular 'codes' which patients can use to alert staff that they wish to speak to them in private (this may be important where a partner or family member accompanies a patient or client to appointments or for treatment). For example, the use of coloured stickers on urine sample bottles is one initiative that has been used. However, if alerts are in place, it is also important to ensure that this information is not made available to perpetrators—this has particular resonance with a recent campaign whereby a 'black dot' marked by a patient on their palm denoted DVA was widely publicised on social media, and as such rendered unsafe and unusable by many commentators.

Time to Reflect
Preparation to identify and respond to DVA is paramount. How well prepared do you feel in this regard and what education and/or training resources are available to you or are you aware of in your area of practice?

Do you have a room in your clinical area where you can speak privately to patients or clients? (Behind curtains or screens is clearly not private or confidential).

In your area of practice, how might patients or clients alert you that they wished to speak with you in private?

10.5 Assessment and Referral Tools

As mentioned earlier, if a patient or client discloses DVA, healthcare professionals may not feel confident to undertake an assessment of risk or know how or where to make a referral for services or support. Moreover, in particular circumstances it will be necessary to liaise and work with other disciplines or services, for example, safeguarding services (Please see Chap. 9). There are a number of different tools to help healthcare professionals assess DVA and in this section an overview of these tools is provided.

A wide range of tools or questionnaires have been developed to screen for DVA more broadly. A systematic review found 18 screening tools for women, many of which were valid and reliable for use in healthcare settings, though none had been tested in the UK (Feder et al. 2009). Common DVA tools reported in the literature include Abuse Assessment Screen (AAS), Composite Abuse Scale (CAS), Humiliation, Afraid, Rape, Kick (HARK), Hurt/Insult/Threaten/Scream (HITS), Parent Screening Questionnaire (PSQ), Partner violence screen (PVS), Woman Abuse Screening Tool (WAST), Women's experience with battering scale (WEB) and Conflicts Tactic Scale-2 (CTS-2). The original CTS was 80 items assessing intra-family conflict and violence; the CTS-2 has 39 items, but each asks about the partici-pant and the partner, making 78 in total; CTS2 has 10 items. Among these various tools, the Hurts, Insults, Threatens and Screams (HITS) scale was the most accurate, with a sensitivity ranging from 86 to 100% and a specificity from 86 to 99% against the reference standard of Index of Spouse Abuse-Physical (ISA-P) plus Woman Abuse Screening Tool (WAST) (Feder et al. 2009). The most commonly used tool in the UK, for example, is the Domestic Abuse, Stalking and Honour Based Violence (DASH) though it is not empirically tested for validity and reliability.

It is important to note, however, that most of these screening instruments are developed and tested in western countries and unless further studies are conducted in other parts of the world, especially in non-developed, eastern and Asian countries to test the usefulness, relevance and applicability of available tools, their applicability is questionable. Definitions and perspective about DVA differ in different cultures and therefore, a need of developing culturally specific tools for different populations and contexts cannot be overlooked. However, in addition to not having a gold stan-dard tool, the available screening tools and their accuracies have not been reviewed in male populations or in couples in same-sex relationships in most countries includ-ing the UK. In addition to the availability of screening instruments, their method of administration is of importance too. There are various screening methods that can be used by healthcare professionals and these include computer based screening, writ-ten or pen and paper screening, audiotape questionnaires, and verbal screening (Svavarsdottir 2010; Hugl-Wajek et al. 2012; Hugl-Wajek et al. 2009; Houry et al. 2008). The effectiveness of any particular screening method may depend on the con-textual factors, such as where it was administered, comfort and confidence of the person using the method and state, willingness, comfort and confidence of the vic-tim-survivor. Some evidence suggests that computer based screening methods are most effective, as victim-survivors can answer questions themselves without being interrupted and therefore convey a sense of confidentiality (Ahmad et al. 2017). On the other hand, verbal screening methods can be most effective if the professional is able to develop a trusting relationship with the victim-survivor. This can help with sensitive inquiry to ensure appropriate information is ascertained and recorded.

Time to Reflect
Within your own area of practice do you currently use a DVA assessment tool? What are your thoughts about its usefulness?

10.6 Gathering Information and Recording

Box 10.1 presents information that should be recorded in notes. As with all aspects of professional record keeping there are key areas to consider when gathering information which may also be utilised for other purposes by other agencies, for example, in criminal proceedings (Department of Health 2017). These include but are not limited to the following:

- Ensure to keep a detailed record of what was discussed with the patient when you suspect DVA. It may be that the patient does not disclose DVA but they might do so in future.
- To ensure confidentiality, records should be accessible to those directly involved in provision of care to victim-survivor.
- Do not record DVA in hand-held notes (e.g. maternity notes).
- You do not need a patient's permission to record a disclosure of DVA or details of your assessment, clinical judgement and examination. It is important to directly communicate to the patient that as part of your duty of care, you are required to keep a record of their disclosure and injuries.

Box 10.1 Information to Record in Notes
Following information should be recorded in the notes:

- Your suspicion of DVA and if it has resulted in (or not) disclosure
- If you have made a routine or selective enquiry and the response
- Detail about perpetrator (relationship, name)
- If the woman is pregnant
- If children live in the same household and age of the children
- Type of abuse experienced (psychological/physical abuse)
- Description of specific recent DVA incidents; duration and frequency of DVA
- Any injuries and specific details
- Presence of increased risk factors
- Results of completed domestic abuse, stalking and honour based violence (DASH) risk assessment for the adult and a domestic violence risk identification matrix (DVRIM) or DASH assessments for each child, if relevant
- Detail of the information provided on local sources of help
- Detail of the action taken (referral)

Adapted from: Department of Health (2017). Responding to domestic abuse: A resource for health professionals. London: Department of Health

- When recording information, describe exactly and clearly what the patient has told you. Use their own words to describe what they have said, using quotation marks.
- Document details of injuries using body maps to show the extent of the injury. Also record the patient's explanation of the injury as well as your findings of your own clinical judgement about consistency between the patient's report and presentation of injuries.
- With consent of the victim-survivor, take photographs and add them onto the notes as a proof of injuries. Ensure to sign and date photographs.
- Explore and record any information or concerns related to DVA on dependent children.
- Ensure that information about DVA is not visible on the opening screen of a patient's record to protect confidentiality.

As DVA victims-survivors are in the healthcare facilities only for a short period of time and will need to be referred to appropriate sources of support outside of healthcare facilities, healthcare organisations should have appropriate policies and pathways delineating identification, management and referral procedures. As a healthcare professional, it is important for you to be aware of the policies, procedure and referral pathways used in the organisation. In addition, information about how to access specialist advice within and outside organisation should be made easily available to those who access services—however, as we have highlighted previously, safety of those experiencing DVA is paramount in all situations.

Time to Reflect
Do you currently have a clear referral pathway for patients and/or clients to other services and support? Do you know what services and supports are available for those who disclose DVA in your area of practice, organisation and locality—and are contact details available to you? Do you know how to make a referral to adult and children's safeguarding services?

Resources to help you
The following resource also lists a number of training resources for healthcare professionals in the UK
  Department of Health (2017) **Responding to Domestic Abuse: A Guide for Healthcare Professionals**
    https://www.gov.uk/government/publications/domestic-abuse-a-resource-for-health-professionals
    The following resource also lists a number of assessment resources for healthcare professionals in the UK
  Department of Health (2017) **Responding to Domestic Abuse: A Guide for Healthcare Professionals**
    https://www.gov.uk/government/publications/domestic-abuse-a-resource-for-health-professionals

10.7 Working with Perpetrators of DVA

In this book, we have not explicitly addressed the particular issues or context surrounding working with perpetrators of DVA. However, the literature in this field is increasingly drawing attention to the importance and necessity of working with perpetrators as well as victim-survivors. For example, Article 16 of The Istanbul Convention[1] describes working with perpetrators both in terms of driving cultural change and in responsibility for actions (Hester and Lilley 2014). As a healthcare professional you may also encounter DVA perpetrators as patients or clients or through a partner or children affected by DVA. How you approach them depends on if they have been identified as abusers by others (victim-survivor), if they directly acknowledge their abusive behaviour as an issue or seek help for a related issue. When engaging with perpetrators, you should consider your own safety and that of the victim-survivor and any children (the particular situation of children and DVA is addressed in detail in Chap. 6). As a healthcare professional, you should be aware of your organisation's policies and referral pathways to any local perpetrator programmes and details of the services offered to DVA perpetrators and we would encourage you to explore this further.

10.8 Chapter Summary and Concluding Comments

In this chapter, we have considered some of the practical issues and next steps for healthcare professionals as they consider DVA within their everyday practice. We hope that you have found this chapter helpful in starting to formulate plans for your own professional and personal development and to consider some of the practicalities of your working environment in supporting disclosure of DVA.

Taken as a whole, the intention of the book is to provide an introduction and overview of some of the key issues surrounding DVA within the particular context of healthcare. We hope that you will use the individual chapters, reflections and resources that we and the chapter authors have included as a starting point for further and more detailed exploration. DVA is a complex phenomenon and a pivotal concern for healthcare professionals and as such forms an important part of contemporary healthcare practice across a range of settings.

10.9 Resources

We have also included three of our recent publications which discuss responding to DVA in different practice contexts:

[1] Domestic and sexual violence perpetrator programmes: Article 16 of the Istanbul Convention https://rm.coe.int/168046e1f2

Ali P, McGarry J (2018) Responding to intimate partner violence in health care settings. Nurs Stand 32(24):54–62

McGarry J, Ali P (2018) Responding to domestic violence and abuse: considerations for health visitors. J Health Visit 6(2):95–98

McGarry J, Carr J (2018) Spotting signs of domestic abuse. Nurs Pract 104:44

Department of Health (2017) Responding to Domestic Abuse: A Guide for Healthcare Professionals https://www.gov.uk/government/publications/domestic-abuse-a-resource-for-health-professionals

Project Mirabel available at: https://www.dur.ac.uk/criva/projectmirabal/

IRIS **http://www.irisdomesticviolence.org.uk/iris/**

References

Ahmad I, Ali PA, Rehman S, Talpur A, Dhingra K (2017) Intimate partner violence screening in emergency department: a rapid review of the literature. J Clin Nurs 26(21–22):3271–3285

Ali P, McGarry J (2018) Supporting people who experience intimate partner violence. Nurs Stand 32(24):54–62

Bradbury-Jones C, Clark M, Taylor J (2017) Abused women's experiences of a primary care identification and referral intervention: a case study analysis. J Adv Nurs 73(12):3189–3199

Department of Health (2017) Responding to domestic abuse: a resource for health professionals. Department of Health, London

Feder G, Ramsay J, Dunne D, Rose M, Arsene C, Norman R, et al (2009) How far does screening women for domestic (partner) violence in different health-care settings meet criteria for a screening programme? Systematic reviews of nine UK National Screening Committee criteria. Health Technol Assess 13(16), iii-iv, xi-xiii, 1–113, 137–347. https://doi.org/10.3310/hta13160

Feder G, Davies RA, Baird K, Dunne D, Eldridge S, Griffiths C, Ramsay J (2011) Identification and Referral to Improve Safety (IRIS) of women experiencing domestic violence with a primary care training and support programme: a cluster randomised controlled trial. Lancet 378(9805):1788–1795

Hester M, Lilley SJ (2014) Domestic and sexual violence perpetrator programmes: article 16 of the Istanbul convention–a collection of papers on the Council of Europe Convention on preventing and combating violence against women and domestic violence. https://rm.coe.int/168046e1f2

Houry D, Kaslow NJ, Kemball RS, McNutt LA, Cerulli C, Straus H et al (2008) Does screening in the emergency department hurt or help victims of intimate partner violence? Ann Emerg Med 51(4):433–442.e437

Hugl-Wajek JA, Cairo D, Shah S, McCreary B (2009) Violence: recognition, management, and prevention. J Emerg Med 2:3–15

Hugl-Wajek JA, Cairo D, Shah S, McCreary B (2012) Detection of domestic violence by a domestic violence advocate in the ED. J Emerg Med 43(5):860–865

Malpass A, Sales K, Johnson M, Howell A, Agnew-Davies R, Feder G (2014) Women's experiences of referral to a domestic violence advocate in UK primary care settings: a service-user collaborative study. Br J Gen Pract 64(620):e151–e158

McGarry J, Hussain B, Watts K (2019) Exploring primary care responses to domestic violence and abuse (DVA): operationalisation of a national initiative. J Adult Prot 21(2):144–154

Safe Lives (2012) Insights into domestic abuse (1). A place of greater safety

Svavarsdottir EK (2010) Detecting intimate partner abuse within clinical settings: self-report or an interview. Scand J Caring Sci 24:224–232

CPI Antony Rowe
Eastbourne, UK
February 06, 2020